from the
Heart of our House

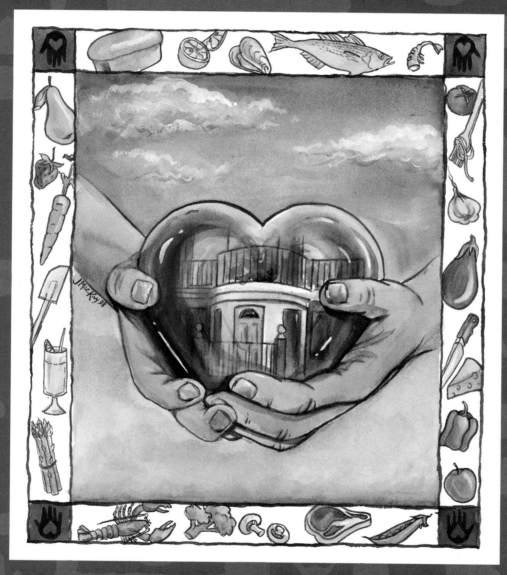

A collection of recipes from the families and friends of the Ronald McDonald House of Providence

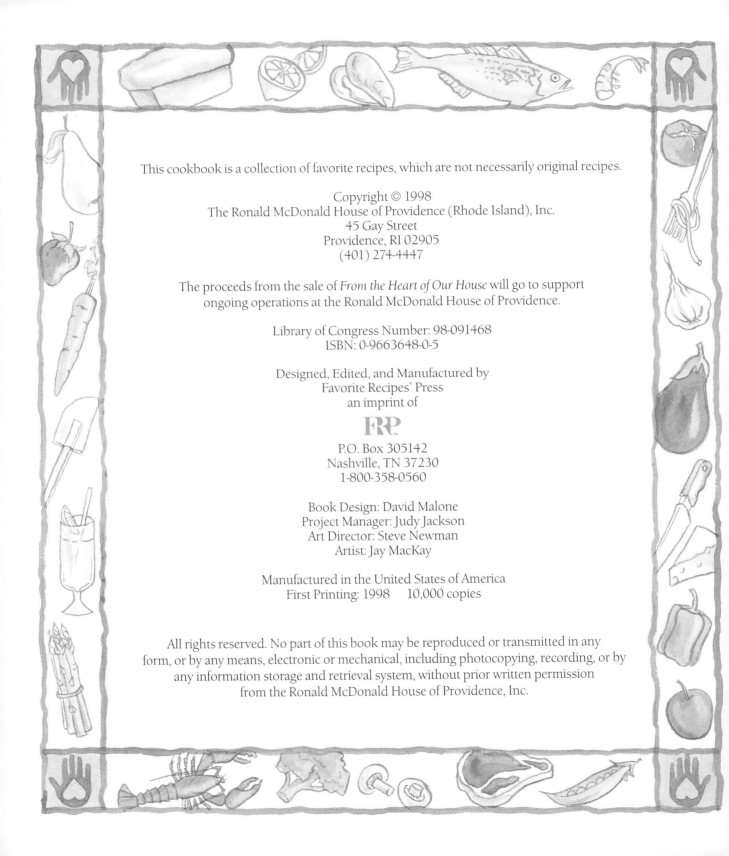

Copyright © 1998
The Ronald McDonald House of Providence (Rhode Island), Inc.
45 Gay Street
Providence, RI 02905
(401) 274-4447

The proceeds from the sale of *From the Heart of Our House* will go to support
ongoing operations at the Ronald McDonald House of Providence.

Library of Congress Number: 98-091468
ISBN: 0-9663648-0-5

Designed, Edited, and Manufactured by
Favorite Recipes® Press
an imprint of

FRP™

P.O. Box 305142
Nashville, TN 37230
1-800-358-0560

Book Design: David Malone
Project Manager: Judy Jackson
Art Director: Steve Newman
Artist: Jay MacKay

Manufactured in the United States of America
First Printing: 1998   10,000 copies

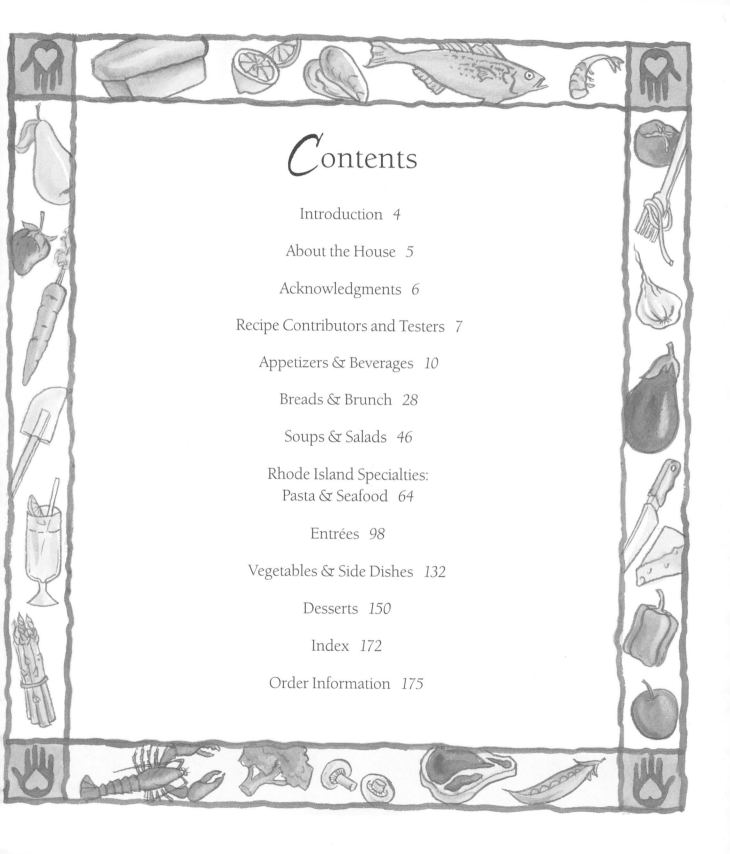

Contents

Introduction 4

About the House 5

Acknowledgments 6

Recipe Contributors and Testers 7

Appetizers & Beverages 10

Breads & Brunch 28

Soups & Salads 46

Rhode Island Specialties:
Pasta & Seafood 64

Entrées 98

Vegetables & Side Dishes 132

Desserts 150

Index 172

Order Information 175

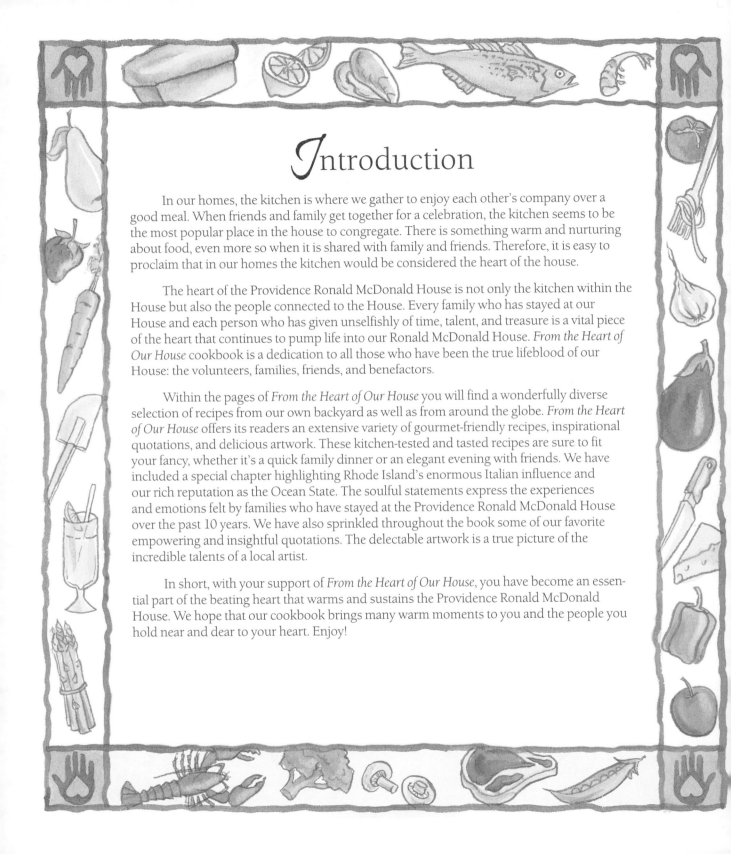

Introduction

In our homes, the kitchen is where we gather to enjoy each other's company over a good meal. When friends and family get together for a celebration, the kitchen seems to be the most popular place in the house to congregate. There is something warm and nurturing about food, even more so when it is shared with family and friends. Therefore, it is easy to proclaim that in our homes the kitchen would be considered the heart of the house.

The heart of the Providence Ronald McDonald House is not only the kitchen within the House but also the people connected to the House. Every family who has stayed at our House and each person who has given unselfishly of time, talent, and treasure is a vital piece of the heart that continues to pump life into our Ronald McDonald House. *From the Heart of Our House* cookbook is a dedication to all those who have been the true lifeblood of our House: the volunteers, families, friends, and benefactors.

Within the pages of *From the Heart of Our House* you will find a wonderfully diverse selection of recipes from our own backyard as well as from around the globe. *From the Heart of Our House* offers its readers an extensive variety of gourmet-friendly recipes, inspirational quotations, and delicious artwork. These kitchen-tested and tasted recipes are sure to fit your fancy, whether it's a quick family dinner or an elegant evening with friends. We have included a special chapter highlighting Rhode Island's enormous Italian influence and our rich reputation as the Ocean State. The soulful statements express the experiences and emotions felt by families who have stayed at the Providence Ronald McDonald House over the past 10 years. We have also sprinkled throughout the book some of our favorite empowering and insightful quotations. The delectable artwork is a true picture of the incredible talents of a local artist.

In short, with your support of *From the Heart of Our House*, you have become an essential part of the beating heart that warms and sustains the Providence Ronald McDonald House. We hope that our cookbook brings many warm moments to you and the people you hold near and dear to your heart. Enjoy!

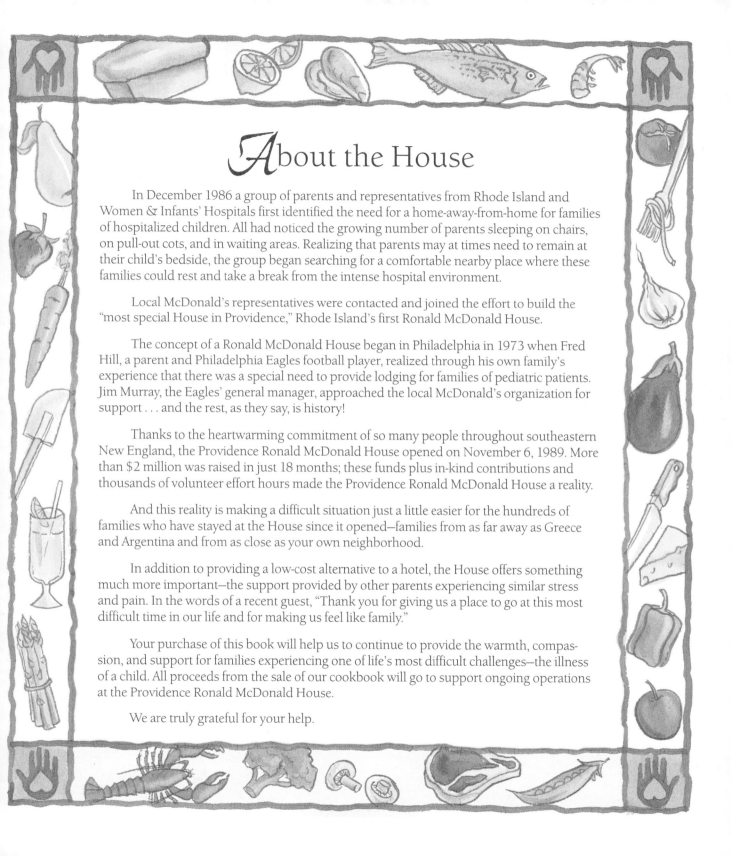

About the House

In December 1986 a group of parents and representatives from Rhode Island and Women & Infants' Hospitals first identified the need for a home-away-from-home for families of hospitalized children. All had noticed the growing number of parents sleeping on chairs, on pull-out cots, and in waiting areas. Realizing that parents may at times need to remain at their child's bedside, the group began searching for a comfortable nearby place where these families could rest and take a break from the intense hospital environment.

Local McDonald's representatives were contacted and joined the effort to build the "most special House in Providence," Rhode Island's first Ronald McDonald House.

The concept of a Ronald McDonald House began in Philadelphia in 1973 when Fred Hill, a parent and Philadelphia Eagles football player, realized through his own family's experience that there was a special need to provide lodging for families of pediatric patients. Jim Murray, the Eagles' general manager, approached the local McDonald's organization for support . . . and the rest, as they say, is history!

Thanks to the heartwarming commitment of so many people throughout southeastern New England, the Providence Ronald McDonald House opened on November 6, 1989. More than $2 million was raised in just 18 months; these funds plus in-kind contributions and thousands of volunteer effort hours made the Providence Ronald McDonald House a reality.

And this reality is making a difficult situation just a little easier for the hundreds of families who have stayed at the House since it opened—families from as far away as Greece and Argentina and from as close as your own neighborhood.

In addition to providing a low-cost alternative to a hotel, the House offers something much more important—the support provided by other parents experiencing similar stress and pain. In the words of a recent guest, "Thank you for giving us a place to go at this most difficult time in our life and for making us feel like family."

Your purchase of this book will help us to continue to provide the warmth, compassion, and support for families experiencing one of life's most difficult challenges—the illness of a child. All proceeds from the sale of our cookbook will go to support ongoing operations at the Providence Ronald McDonald House.

We are truly grateful for your help.

$\mathcal{A}$cknowledgments

Cookbook Committee

Carol M. Barnabe, Co-chair
Margaret Gardner, Co-chair
Gail Fraser-Giacchi
Carolyn Killian

Jay MacKay
Mary E. McGinn
Gail Rubenstein
Janice Santucci

We want to give special thanks to Carolyn Killian, co-chair of a Tabasco Award-winning cookbook, whose help has been invaluable to our project.

A special thank you to Mary McGinn for her time and efforts in making this book possible.

Artist Jay MacKay received his BFA from the University of Lowell and has continued his studies at the Worcester Art Museum and the DeCordova Museum. We are very grateful to this talented local artist for his generous gift of all artwork in our book.

We could not have produced this cookbook without the support and friendship of the staff, faculty, and students of Johnson & Wales University, in particular Pamela Peters, director of culinary education; Michael Marra, associate professor, Food Service Academics Department; and Frank Terranova, certified executive chef.

The generous support of the following major sponsors has also proved essential in the production of *From the Heart of Our House*.

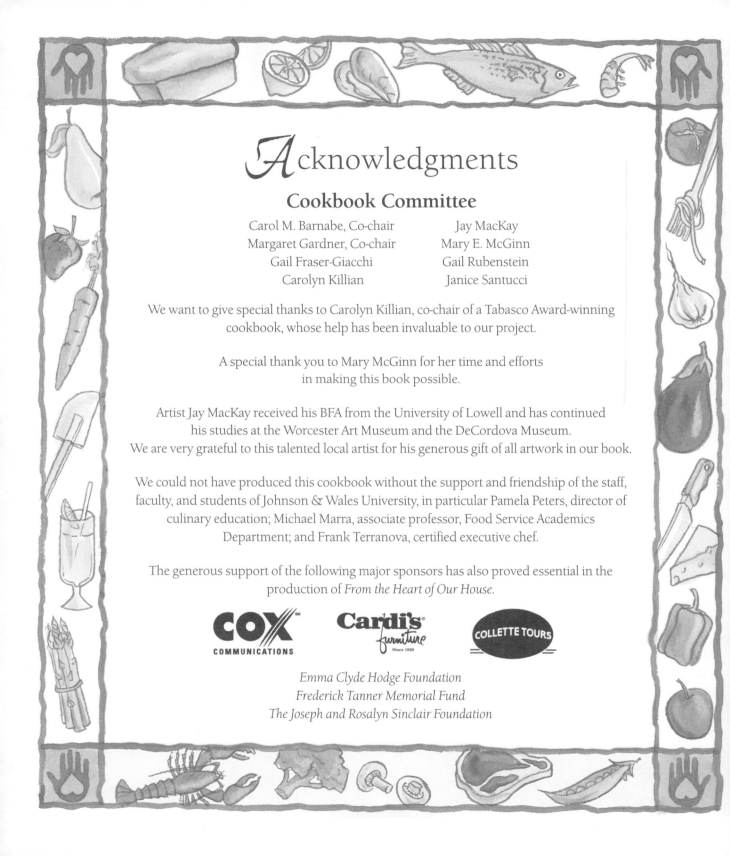

Emma Clyde Hodge Foundation
Frederick Tanner Memorial Fund
The Joseph and Rosalyn Sinclair Foundation

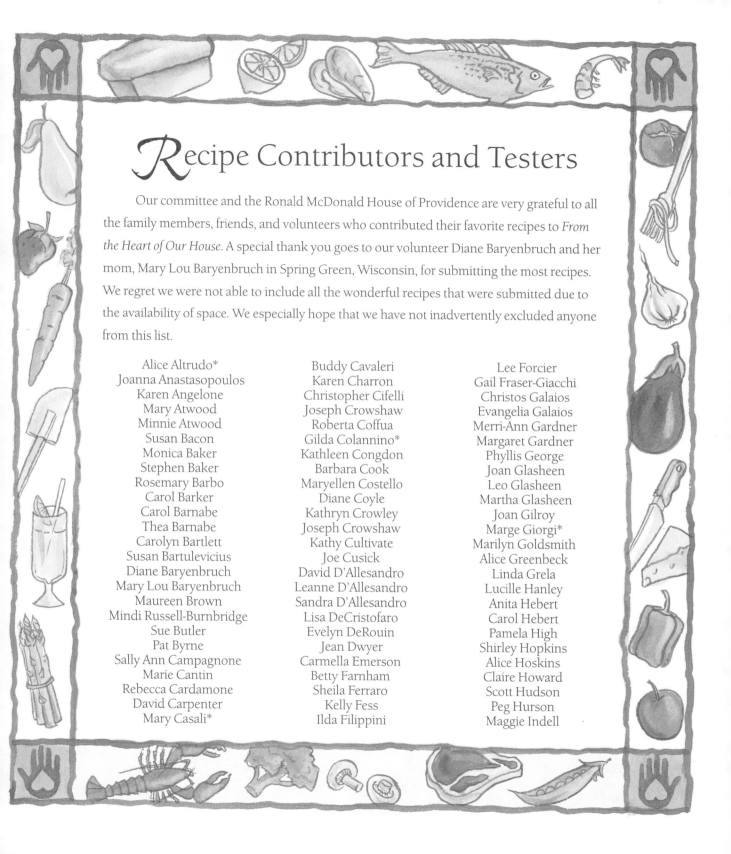

Recipe Contributors and Testers

Our committee and the Ronald McDonald House of Providence are very grateful to all the family members, friends, and volunteers who contributed their favorite recipes to *From the Heart of Our House*. A special thank you goes to our volunteer Diane Baryenbruch and her mom, Mary Lou Baryenbruch in Spring Green, Wisconsin, for submitting the most recipes. We regret we were not able to include all the wonderful recipes that were submitted due to the availability of space. We especially hope that we have not inadvertently excluded anyone from this list.

Alice Altrudo*
Joanna Anastasopoulos
Karen Angelone
Mary Atwood
Minnie Atwood
Susan Bacon
Monica Baker
Stephen Baker
Rosemary Barbo
Carol Barker
Carol Barnabe
Thea Barnabe
Carolyn Bartlett
Susan Bartulevicius
Diane Baryenbruch
Mary Lou Baryenbruch
Maureen Brown
Mindi Russell-Burnbridge
Sue Butler
Pat Byrne
Sally Ann Campagnone
Marie Cantin
Rebecca Cardamone
David Carpenter
Mary Casali*

Buddy Cavaleri
Karen Charron
Christopher Cifelli
Joseph Crowshaw
Roberta Coffua
Gilda Colannino*
Kathleen Congdon
Barbara Cook
Maryellen Costello
Diane Coyle
Kathryn Crowley
Joseph Crowshaw
Kathy Cultivate
Joe Cusick
David D'Allesandro
Leanne D'Allesandro
Sandra D'Allesandro
Lisa DeCristofaro
Evelyn DeRouin
Jean Dwyer
Carmella Emerson
Betty Farnham
Sheila Ferraro
Kelly Fess
Ilda Filippini

Lee Forcier
Gail Fraser-Giacchi
Christos Galaios
Evangelia Galaios
Merri-Ann Gardner
Margaret Gardner
Phyllis George
Joan Glasheen
Leo Glasheen
Martha Glasheen
Joan Gilroy
Marge Giorgi*
Marilyn Goldsmith
Alice Greenbeck
Linda Grela
Lucille Hanley
Anita Hebert
Carol Hebert
Pamela High
Shirley Hopkins
Alice Hoskins
Claire Howard
Scott Hudson
Peg Hurson
Maggie Indell

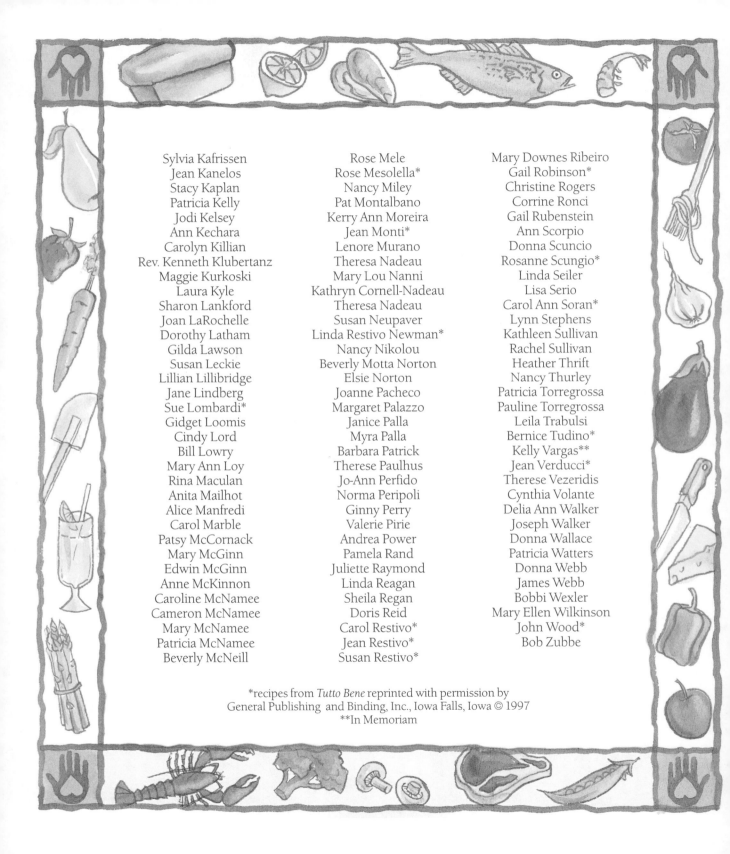

Sylvia Kafrissen
Jean Kanelos
Stacy Kaplan
Patricia Kelly
Jodi Kelsey
Ann Kechara
Carolyn Killian
Rev. Kenneth Klubertanz
Maggie Kurkoski
Laura Kyle
Sharon Lankford
Joan LaRochelle
Dorothy Latham
Gilda Lawson
Susan Leckie
Lillian Lillibridge
Jane Lindberg
Sue Lombardi*
Gidget Loomis
Cindy Lord
Bill Lowry
Mary Ann Loy
Rina Maculan
Anita Mailhot
Alice Manfredi
Carol Marble
Patsy McCornack
Mary McGinn
Edwin McGinn
Anne McKinnon
Caroline McNamee
Cameron McNamee
Mary McNamee
Patricia McNamee
Beverly McNeill

Rose Mele
Rose Mesolella*
Nancy Miley
Pat Montalbano
Kerry Ann Moreira
Jean Monti*
Lenore Murano
Theresa Nadeau
Mary Lou Nanni
Kathryn Cornell-Nadeau
Theresa Nadeau
Susan Neupaver
Linda Restivo Newman*
Nancy Nikolou
Beverly Motta Norton
Elsie Norton
Joanne Pacheco
Margaret Palazzo
Janice Palla
Myra Palla
Barbara Patrick
Therese Paulhus
Jo-Ann Perfido
Norma Peripoli
Ginny Perry
Valerie Pirie
Andrea Power
Pamela Rand
Juliette Raymond
Linda Reagan
Sheila Regan
Doris Reid
Carol Restivo*
Jean Restivo*
Susan Restivo*

Mary Downes Ribeiro
Gail Robinson*
Christine Rogers
Corrine Ronci
Gail Rubenstein
Ann Scorpio
Donna Scuncio
Rosanne Scungio*
Linda Seiler
Lisa Serio
Carol Ann Soran*
Lynn Stephens
Kathleen Sullivan
Rachel Sullivan
Heather Thrift
Nancy Thurley
Patricia Torregrossa
Pauline Torregrossa
Leila Trabulsi
Bernice Tudino*
Kelly Vargas**
Jean Verducci*
Therese Vezeridis
Cynthia Volante
Delia Ann Walker
Joseph Walker
Donna Wallace
Patricia Watters
Donna Webb
James Webb
Bobbi Wexler
Mary Ellen Wilkinson
John Wood*
Bob Zubbe

*recipes from *Tutto Bene* reprinted with permission by
General Publishing and Binding, Inc., Iowa Falls, Iowa © 1997
**In Memoriam

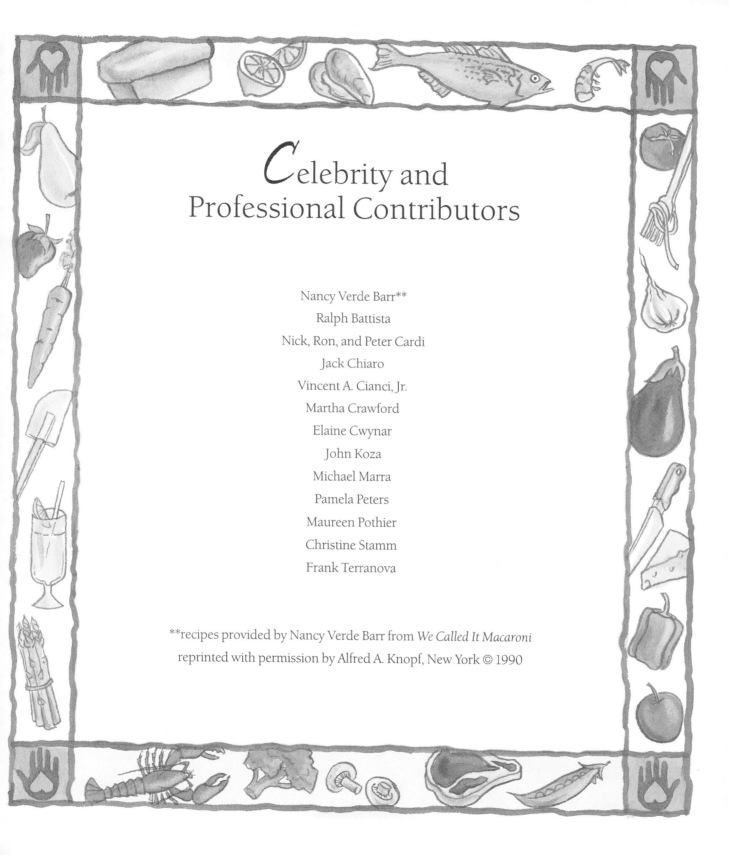

Celebrity and Professional Contributors

Nancy Verde Barr**

Ralph Battista

Nick, Ron, and Peter Cardi

Jack Chiaro

Vincent A. Cianci, Jr.

Martha Crawford

Elaine Cwynar

John Koza

Michael Marra

Pamela Peters

Maureen Pothier

Christine Stamm

Frank Terranova

**recipes provided by Nancy Verde Barr from *We Called It Macaroni*

reprinted with permission by Alfred A. Knopf, New York © 1990

Appetizers & Beverages

"You have opened your door and hearts to countless families throughout the years. This year, by the grace of God, my family and I would also walk through these doors, to be met with open arms and loving hearts. You've given strength when I was weak, hope when I was feeling hopeless, but most of all, love when love is what I needed most."

—Kim Gonzales, parent

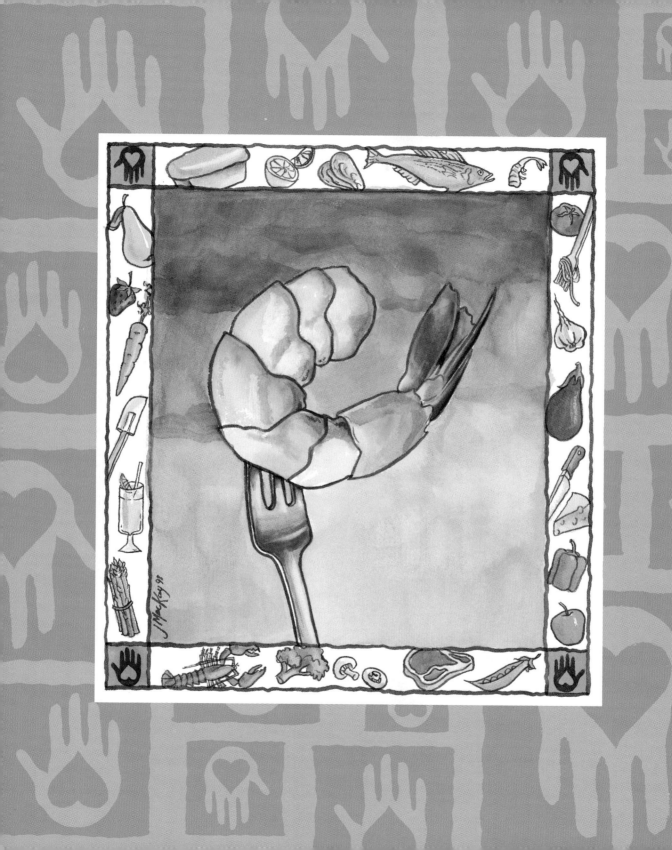

$\mathcal{A}$ppetizers & Beverages

Hot Artichoke Dip 13

Mustard Dill Dip 13

Crab Dip 14

Hummus-Style Dip 15

Herbed Cream Cheese 16

Hot Fresh Salsa 16

Swiss Cheese Spread 17

Olive Nut Spread 17

Baked Brie and Brandied Mushrooms 18

Apple Pizza 19

Asparagus Treats 19

Clams Casino 20

Pepperoni and Cheese Puffs 20

Chile Pepper Pie 20

Vegetable Squares 21

Southwest Appetizer Cheesecake 22

Lemon Chicken 23

Mushroom Palmiers 24

Mint Cooler 25

Raspberry Slush 25

Sophisticated Strawberry Shakes 26

Strawberry Smoothie 26

Old New England Hot Mulled Punch 27

Hot Buttered Sherry 27

Hot Artichoke Dip

2 (14-ounce) cans artichoke
hearts, drained, chopped
1 cup grated Parmesan cheese
1 cup shredded mozzarella cheese

1 cup mayonnaise
1 teaspoon salt
1 clove of garlic, minced

Combine the artichoke hearts, Parmesan cheese, mozzarella cheese, mayonnaise, salt and garlic in a large bowl and mix well. Spoon into a buttered 1½-quart casserole. Bake at 350 degrees for 25 to 30 minutes or until heated through. Serve hot with crackers.

Yield: 30 servings

Mustard Dill Dip

2 tablespoons Dijon mustard
1 tablespoon white wine vinegar
1½ tablespoons sugar

¼ cup chopped fresh dillweed
½ cup light olive oil or vegetable oil

Whisk the Dijon mustard, vinegar, sugar and dillweed in a bowl. Add the olive oil gradually, whisking constantly until the mixture is blended and slightly thickened. Adjust the flavors to taste. Serve with bite-size fresh vegetables and cooked shrimp or as a sauce atop smoked salmon.

Yield: 10 to 15 servings

Crab Dip

8 ounces cream cheese, softened
1/2 cup sherry, brandy, white
wine or chicken broth
1 cup shredded Cheddar cheese
1 teaspoon cornstarch
8 ounces crab meat, flaked, or
imitation crab meat

2 tablespoons finely chopped
parsley or dillweed
1 tablespoon Worcestershire sauce
2 tablespoons half-and-half
Paprika to taste

Combine the cream cheese and sherry in a saucepan. Cook over low heat until the cream cheese is melted, stirring constantly until creamy.

Add the Cheddar cheese, cornstarch, crab meat, parsley, Worcestershire sauce and half-and-half to the cream cheese mixture and mix well. Cook over medium-low heat until hot, stirring frequently; do not boil.

Spoon the mixture into a hot chafing dish or fondue pot. Sprinkle with paprika. Serve warm with white toast triangles, chips, celery sticks, green bell pepper strips or green peas.

Yield: 15 servings

From the Heart...

"Nothing can replace the shock of pleasure given by a small mountain of fresh basil in the summer kitchen."
—Eleanor Perenyi

...of Our House

Hummus-Style Dip

1 (19-ounce) can chick-peas,
drained, rinsed
Juice of $1/2$ lemon
1 clove of garlic, chopped
$1/8$ teaspoon cayenne, or to taste
2 tablespoons (or more) water

1 tablespoon extra-virgin olive oil
1 tablespoon chopped mint
1 tablespoon chopped
flat-leaf parsley
1 tablespoon chopped dillweed

Combine the chick-peas, lemon juice, garlic, cayenne and 2 tablespoons water in a food processor container. Process at high speed until the mixture is puréed, adding more water if needed to make a smooth paste. Drizzle in the olive oil with the food processor running. Add the mint, parsley and dillweed. Pulse briefly until blended.

Serve in a crock, ramekin or bowl surrounded by cut pita bread, French bread and/or bite-size fresh vegetables.

Editor's Note: Use your creativity to vary this recipe to your own taste. Some suggestions include: omit the mint and dillweed and add 1 tablespoon fresh basil and 1 chopped seeded tomato; add 6 black or green olives when you add the herbs, leaving the olives slightly chunky for texture; omit the dillweed and mint and add 2 tablespoons medium or hot salsa; or stir in $1/4$ cup thawed frozen chopped spinach (squeezed dry) and 1 tablespoon crumbled feta cheese. You may also replace the chick-peas with other canned beans, but then the dip will not taste like hummus.

Yield: 15 to 20 servings

$\mathcal{H}$erbed Cream Cheese

8 ounces cream cheese, softened
4 ounces whipped unsalted butter
1 clove of garlic, crushed
1/8 teaspoon pepper
1/8 teaspoon thyme

1/8 teaspoon basil
1/8 teaspoon marjoram
1/8 teaspoon dillweed
1/8 teaspoon oregano

Combine the cream cheese, butter, garlic, pepper, thyme, basil, marjoram, dillweed and oregano in a bowl and mix well. Chill, covered, for 24 hours. Let stand at room temperature until softened before serving. Serve with crackers or bagel chips.

Yield: 4 servings

$\mathcal{H}$ot Fresh Salsa

1 (4-ounce) can sliced
black olives, drained
1 (4-ounce) can chopped green chiles
1 onion, chopped
2 tomatoes, chopped

1 1/2 tablespoons white vinegar
3 tablespoons olive oil
1 1/2 teaspoons garlic salt
Chopped fresh cilantro to taste

Mix the olives, undrained chiles, onion, tomatoes, vinegar, olive oil, garlic salt and cilantro in a bowl. Chill, covered, until serving time. Serve with tortilla chips.

Editor's Note: Vary the flavor of this salsa by decreasing the amount of vinegar and adjusting the amount of green chiles to your own taste.

Yield: 30 servings

Swiss Cheese Spread

1 (8-ounce) package shredded
Swiss cheese
10 ounces cream cheese, softened

1 cup mayonnaise
1/2 cup chopped onion

Mix the Swiss cheese, cream cheese, mayonnaise and onion in a bowl. Spread in a 6x10-inch baking dish. Bake at 400 degrees for 10 minutes. Serve with bite-size crackers. May be prepared with low-fat or nonfat cheeses and mayonnaise.

Yield: 40 servings

Olive Nut Spread

1/2 cup plus 2 tablespoons
chopped salad olives
8 ounces cream cheese, softened
1/2 cup plus 2 tablespoons mayonnaise

1/2 cup plus 2 tablespoons
chopped pecans
1/8 teaspoon pepper, or to taste

Drain the olives, reserving 2 tablespoons of the liquid. Mix the cream cheese, mayonnaise, pecans, olives, reserved liquid and pepper in a bowl. Chill, covered, for 24 hours. Serve on crostini, crackers or cocktail rye bread.

Yield: 20 to 30 servings

Baked Brie and Brandied Mushrooms

1 tablespoon margarine or butter
2 tablespoons slivered almonds
1 cup chopped fresh mushrooms
2 cloves of garlic, minced
1 tablespoon brandy

1 teaspoon chopped fresh tarragon, or
1/4 teaspoon dried
1/8 teaspoon pepper
1 (8-ounce) round Brie

Melt the margarine in a medium skillet over medium heat. Add the almonds. Cook for 2 to 3 minutes or until the almonds are browned, stirring constantly.

Stir in the mushrooms, garlic, brandy, tarragon and pepper. Cook for 1 to 2 minutes or until the mushrooms are tender, stirring constantly. Remove from the heat.

Place the cheese in a decorative shallow baking dish or an 8- or 9-inch round baking dish. Spoon the mushroom mixture over the top.

Bake at 375 degrees for 10 to 12 minutes or until the cheese is soft. Garnish with 2 sprigs of fresh tarragon. Serve with melba toast rounds or crackers.

Yield: 16 servings

From the Heart...

"Think this over carefully; the most charming hours of our life are all connected—by a more or less tangible hyphen—with a memory of the table."
—Pierre-Charles Monselet

...of Our House

Apple Pizza

Prepared pizza dough for 1 pizza
Melted butter
4 to 5 apples, peeled, cored, sliced

1 (8-ounce) package shredded
mozzarella cheese
2 teaspoons cinnamon
1/2 cup sugar

Spread the pizza dough over a greased round or oblong pizza pan. Spread a small amount of melted butter over the dough. Arrange the apples in a single layer over the dough. Sprinkle with the cheese. Top with a mixture of the cinnamon and sugar. Bake at 350 degrees until the crust is browned.

Yield: 8 to 12 servings

Asparagus Treats

1 loaf thinly sliced white bread,
crusts trimmed
4 ounces cream cheese, softened
4 ounces Roquefort cheese or bleu
cheese, crumbled
1 tablespoon mayonnaise

1 egg, beaten
1 (15-ounce) can asparagus
spears, drained
Melted butter
Paprika to taste

Flatten each bread slice with a rolling pin. Mix the cream cheese, Roquefort cheese, mayonnaise and egg in a bowl. Spread over the bread slices. Top each with 1 asparagus spear and roll up. Cut each roll into 2 to 3 pieces. Brush each with melted butter. Sprinkle with paprika. Place the rolls on a baking sheet. Bake at 350 degrees for 15 minutes. May substitute puff pastry for the bread. May freeze before baking.

Yield: 15 to 20 servings

Clams Casino

24 cherrystone clams
1/4 cup butter or margarine
1 large clove of garlic, finely chopped

2 teaspoons chopped pimentos
3/4 cup Italian bread crumbs

Open the clams and discard the tops; set the clams aside. Melt the butter in a saucepan. Add the garlic. Sauté until tender. Add the pimentos and bread crumbs and mix well. Top each clam with approximately 1 teaspoon of the pimento mixture. Place the clams in a baking pan. Bake at 450 degrees for 10 minutes.

Yield: 4 to 6 servings

Pepperoni and Cheese Puffs

2 to 4 pounds Italian dough
1 (8-ounce) can tomato sauce
2 packages extra-sharp Cheddar
cheese, sliced

1 stick pepperoni, sliced
Vegetable oil

Cut the dough into 3x4-inch pieces. Place 1/2 teaspoon tomato sauce in the center of each piece. Top each with cheese and pepperoni slices. Press the corners of each dough piece together tightly and seal. Place sealed side down on a lightly greased pizza pan. Repeat with the remaining dough pieces. Brush the tops with vegetable oil. Bake at 450 degrees for 15 minutes or until the tops are browned.

Yield: 24 to 48 servings

Chile Pepper Pie

2 (4-ounce) cans chopped
green chiles, drained
10 ounces Cheddar cheese, shredded

2 eggs
2 tablespoons milk

Place the green chiles in an 8x8-inch baking pan. Sprinkle evenly with the cheese. Beat the eggs and milk in a small bowl. Spoon the egg mixture over the chiles. Bake at 350 degrees for 1 hour. Cool slightly before cutting into 1x1-inch pieces.

Yield: 64 servings

Vegetable Squares

1 (8-ounce) package croissant dough
3 tablespoons cream cheese, softened
1 tablespoon mayonnaise
1 teaspoon garlic powder

$^{1}/_{2}$ cup blanched broccoli florets
$^{1}/_{2}$ cup shredded carrot
$^{1}/_{2}$ cup chopped green bell pepper
$^{1}/_{2}$ cup chopped red bell pepper

Spread the croissant dough in a greased 8x10-inch baking pan. Bake at 350 degrees for 15 minutes or until golden brown. Let cool. Mix the cream cheese, mayonnaise and garlic powder in a bowl. Spread over the baked crust. Top with the broccoli, carrot and bell peppers. Chill, covered, until serving time. Cut into squares. You may use low-fat cream cheese and mayonnaise in this recipe.

Yield: 20 servings

Southwest Appetizer Cheesecake

1⅓ cups finely crushed tortilla chips
¼ cup melted butter
1 cup cottage cheese
24 ounces cream cheese, softened
4 eggs
2 cups shredded Cheddar cheese
1 (4-ounce) can chopped
green chiles, drained

1 cup sour cream
1 (8-ounce) package jalapeño
cheese dip
1 cup chopped tomato
½ cup chopped green onions
¼ cup sliced black olives

Combine the tortilla chip crumbs and butter in a bowl and mix well. Press over the bottom of a 10-inch springform pan. Bake at 325 degrees for 15 minutes.

Process the cottage cheese in a blender at high speed until smooth. Combine the cottage cheese and cream cheese in a mixer bowl and beat until blended.

Add the eggs 1 at a time to the cheese mixture, beating well after each addition. Stir in the Cheddar cheese and green chiles. Spoon over the crust. Bake at 325 degrees for 50 minutes.

Combine the sour cream and cheese dip in a bowl and mix well. Spread over the green chile mixture. Bake for 10 minutes longer.

Loosen the cheesecake from the rim of the pan. Cool completely before removing the side of the pan. Chill until serving time. Top with the tomato, green onions and sliced olives. Serve with favorite crackers, chips or bite-size fresh vegetables.

Yield: 20 to 24 servings

Lemon Chicken

1 cup flour
2 teaspoons salt
1/4 teaspoon pepper
2 teaspoons crumbled sage
1 teaspoon paprika

12 small boneless skinless
chicken breast halves
1/4 cup butter
1/4 cup vegetable oil
Lemon Dressing

Mix the flour, salt, pepper, sage and paprika in a sealable plastic bag. Add the chicken and shake to coat. Heat the butter and oil in a large skillet over medium heat until the butter is melted. Add the chicken a few pieces at a time. Sauté until the chicken is browned and cooked through. Let cool.

Cut each chicken piece into halves lengthwise, then into 4 long strips. Place in a shallow baking dish. Pour Lemon Dressing over the chicken. Marinate, covered, in the refrigerator until serving time.

Yield: 12 to 15 servings

Lemon Dressing

1 cup vegetable oil
2 tablespoons grated lemon peel
1/2 cup lemon juice
1/4 cup sugar

1 teaspoon salt
1/4 teaspoon pepper
2 tablespoons chopped chives

Combine the oil, lemon peel, lemon juice, sugar, salt, pepper and chives in a jar with a tight-fitting lid; cover. Shake well to mix thoroughly.

Mushroom Palmiers

10 slices bread
8 ounces chopped mushrooms
1 small onion, chopped

2 tablespoons butter
8 ounces cream cheese, softened
1/2 cup melted butter

Trim the crusts from the bread. Flatten each bread slice with a rolling pin. Sauté the mushrooms and onion in 2 tablespoons butter in a skillet until the vegetables are tender.

Combine the mushroom mixture and cream cheese in a bowl and mix well. Spread over the bread slices, leaving a small margin at the edges. Roll up as for jelly rolls, pressing to seal the edges.

Dip each roll into the melted butter. Place on a baking sheet and freeze for several hours. Wrap the frozen rolls in plastic wrap or place them in a sealable plastic bag. Store in the refrigerator until baking time. Cut each roll into thirds. Place on a baking sheet. Bake at 400 degrees for 20 minutes.

Yield: 10 servings

From the Heart...

"... the kitchen, the house's warm heart."
–Anne Rivers Siddon

...of Our House

Mint Cooler

1 quart boiling water
2 tablespoons black tea leaves
2 tablespoons chopped fresh mint
2 (750-ml) bottles red wine

½ cup lemon juice
1 cup honey
1 quart sparkling water

Pour the boiling water over the tea leaves in a large container. Steep for 5 minutes. Strain the liquid into a punch bowl. Let cool. Add the wine, lemon juice, honey, sparkling water and ice and mix gently. Add additional honey or sugar if desired. Garnish with fresh lemon slices pierced with sprigs of fresh mint.

Yield: 20 to 30 servings

Raspberry Slush

1 (46-ounce) can pineapple juice
2 (12-ounce) cans frozen lemonade
concentrate, thawed
½ bottle lemon juice
3 envelopes raspberry drink mix

4 cups sugar
1 quart vodka
4 quarts water
Lemon-lime soda or ginger ale

Mix the pineapple juice, lemonade concentrate, lemon juice, drink mix and sugar in a large container. Add the vodka and water and mix well. Divide the mixture evenly between 2 ice cream freezer containers. Freeze until firm, stirring once an hour. To serve, scoop the desired amount into a glass and fill with lemon-lime soda or ginger ale.

Yield: 40 to 50 servings

Sophisticated Strawberry Shakes

1 cup sliced strawberries, chilled
1/2 cup sugar
salt to taste
1 egg, beaten

1 cup cold milk
1 tablespoon cold lemon juice
2/3 cup cold burgundy or
other red wine

Combine the strawberries, sugar, salt, egg and milk in a blender container. Process until smooth. Stir in the lemon juice and wine. Pour into glasses and serve immediately.

Yield: 4 servings

Strawberry Smoothie

1 1/2 cups strawberries, hulled,
cut into halves
2 medium bananas, frozen,
cut into pieces

8 ice cubes
1/2 cup vanilla nonfat yogurt
1 tablespoon honey

Combine the strawberries, bananas, ice cubes, yogurt and honey in a blender container. Process until smooth. Pour into glasses and serve immediately.

Yield: 4 servings

Old New England Hot Mulled Punch

1 cup sugar
1/2 cup water
2 cinnamon sticks
1/2 lemon, sliced

24 whole cloves
4 cups hot orange grapefruit juice
1 quart claret
Brandy to taste

Combine the sugar, water, cinnamon sticks, lemon slices and cloves in a saucepan. Boil for 5 to 10 minutes or until the mixture is heated through and the flavors have blended. Strain through a sieve. Add the grapefruit juice, claret and brandy and mix gently. Serve hot.

Yield: 8 to 12 servings

Hot Buttered Sherry

1 (6-ounce) can any flavor frozen
juice concentrate, thawed
3/4 cup dry sherry
2 1/2 cups water
1 tablespoon sugar

1/4 teaspoon ground cinnamon
1/8 teaspoon salt, or to taste
Softened butter
Cinnamon sticks

Combine the juice concentrate, sherry, water, sugar, cinnamon and salt in a saucepan and mix well. Heat to just below the boiling point. Ladle into mugs. Top each serving with a dollop of butter. Add a cinnamon stick to each mug to use as a stirrer.

Yield: 6 to 8 servings

Breads & Brunch

"It was important to give parents an opportunity to get some rest when they needed it, not to feel guilty about having to leave. One parent could stay with the child while the other could get a few hours' sleep. It's important that the family stay intact as much as possible so that they're available to be supportive to the child who is being cared for."

—Richard Cantin, parent

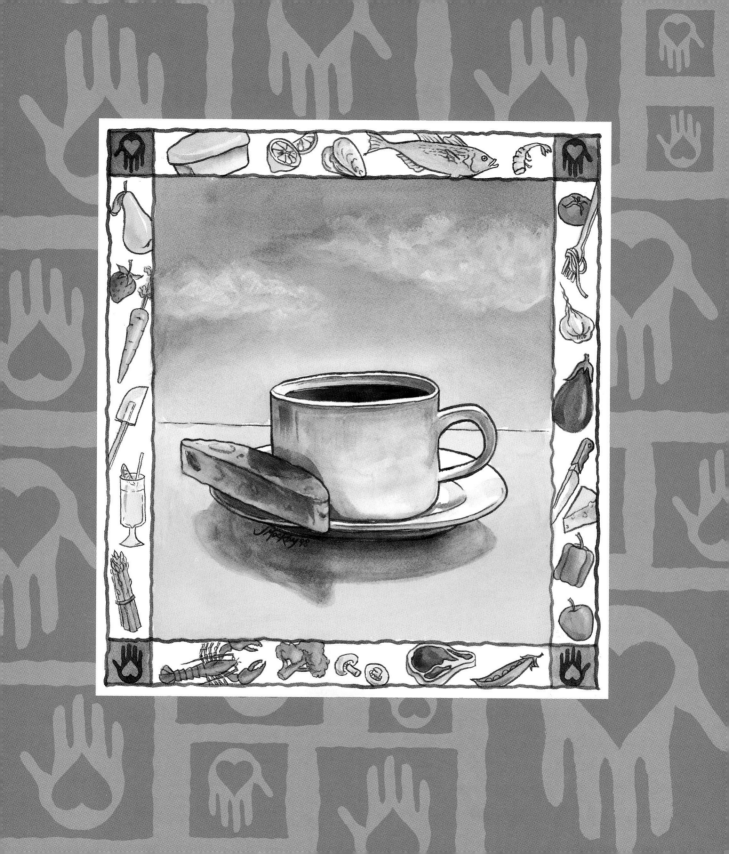

Breads & Brunch

Blueberry Tea Cake 31

New England Brown Bread 32

Garlic Bread 32

Lemon Bread 33

Nirope Nut Bread 34

Strawberry Brunch Loaf 35

Bran Muffins 36

Banana Buttermilk Buckwheat Pancakes 37

Crepes Stuffed with Ricotta Cheese and Prosciutto 38

Biscotti 39

Company Eggs 40

Eggs Rustica 40

Spinach Frittata 41

Sherried Crab Quiche 42

Creamed Lobster and Johnnycakes 43

Shrimp with Creamy Dill Sauce 44

Tomato Mozzarella Tart 45

$\mathcal{B}$lueberry Tea Cake

¹/₄ cup butter or margarine, softened
³/₄ cup sugar
1 egg
2 cups flour
2 teaspoons baking powder
¹/₂ teaspoon salt

¹/₂ cup milk
2 cups blueberries
¹/₂ cup sugar
¹/₄ cup flour
¹/₂ teaspoon cinnamon
¹/₄ cup butter, softened

Combine ¹/₄ cup butter, ³/₄ cup sugar and egg in a large bowl and mix well. Add 2 cups flour, baking powder and salt and mix well. Add the milk and blueberries, stirring gently until mixed.

Spoon the batter into a tube pan sprayed with nonstick cooking spray. Mix ¹/₂ cup sugar, ¹/₄ cup flour, cinnamon and ¹/₄ cup butter in a bowl until crumbly. Sprinkle over the batter.

Bake at 375 degrees for 45 minutes. Cool in the pan for several minutes. Invert onto a serving plate to cool completely.

Yield: 10 to 12 servings

From the Heart...

"When you have a party at home, no matter how much room you have, the guests will automatically manage to work their way into the kitchen . . . warmth and food and life."
—Mary Higgins Clark

...of Our House

New England Brown Bread

3/4 cup honey
3/4 cup molasses
3 1/2 cups flour
2 teaspoons baking soda
2 teaspoons ginger
2 teaspoons cinnamon

2 teaspoons allspice
1/8 teaspoon salt, or to taste
2 cups milk
1 cup raisins
2 tablespoons orange marmalade

Mix the honey and molasses in a bowl. Add the flour, baking soda, ginger, cinnamon, allspice, salt, milk, raisins and marmalade, stirring just until mixed. Spoon into a large buttered baking dish. Bake at 350 degrees for 1 1/4 hours.

Yield: 8 to 10 servings

Garlic Bread

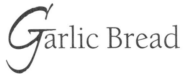

1/4 cup butter, softened
3 cloves of garlic, crushed

1/4 cup shredded Gouda cheese
8 (1/2-inch) slices Italian bread

Mix the butter, garlic and cheese in a bowl. Spread over the bread slices. Place on a baking sheet. Bake at 350 degrees until lightly browned.

Yield: 4 servings

Lemon Bread

1¹/₂ cups sugar
1 cup vegetable oil
Grated peel of 2 lemons
6 eggs
1¹/₃ cups flour

¹/₂ teaspoon salt
2 teaspoons baking powder
¹/₂ to 1 cup floured chopped pecans or
walnuts (optional)
Lemon Glaze

Grease 3 small bread pans and line with waxed paper. Combine the sugar, oil and lemon peel in a bowl and mix well. Add the eggs 1 at a time, beating well after each addition. Add the flour, salt, baking powder and pecans and mix well.

Spoon the batter into the prepared pans. Bake at 300 to 325 degrees for 55 to 60 minutes or until the loaves test done. Spoon Lemon Glaze over the warm bread.

Yield: 24 servings

Lemon Glaze

1 cup confectioners' sugar

Juice of 1 to 2 lemons

Place the confectioners' sugar in a bowl. Add enough lemon juice to make of glaze consistency, stirring until smooth.

Nirope Nut Bread

2½ cups flour
2 teaspoons baking soda
½ teaspoon ground cloves
1½ teaspoons cinnamon
1 teaspoon salt
1 teaspoon baking powder

¾ cup vegetable oil
3 eggs
1½ cups sugar
1 teaspoon vanilla extract
1 cup chopped walnuts
2 cups grated unpeeled zucchini

Sift the flour, baking soda, cloves, cinnamon, salt and baking powder into a small bowl. Combine the oil, eggs and sugar in a mixer bowl, beating until smooth. Add the flour mixture gradually, beating well after each addition. Stir in the vanilla, walnuts and zucchini.

Spoon the batter into a 5x9-inch loaf pan sprayed with nonstick cooking spray. Bake at 350 degrees for 1¼ hours or until a wooden pick inserted near the center comes out clean.

Cool in the pan for several minutes. Loosen the bread from the sides of the pan. Remove to a wire rack to cool completely. Cut into ½-inch slices.

Yield: 10 servings

Strawberry Brunch Loaf

2 cups flour
1 tablespoon baking powder
1 teaspoon salt
2 teaspoons grated lemon peel
1/2 teaspoon nutmeg
2 eggs, beaten

1/2 cup honey
1/2 cup vegetable oil
1 1/2 cups coarsely chopped
strawberries
1/2 cup slivered almonds

Combine the flour, baking powder, salt, lemon peel and nutmeg in a large bowl and mix well. Beat the eggs, honey and oil in a medium bowl. Stir in the strawberries and almonds.

Add the strawberry mixture to the flour mixture, stirring just until moistened. Spoon into a greased 5x9-inch loaf pan.

Bake at 350 degrees for 50 to 55 minutes or until the loaf tests done. Cool in the pan for 15 minutes. Remove to a wire rack to cool completely. Cut into 3/4-inch slices.

Yield: 12 servings

Bran Muffins

2¾ cups sugar
5 cups flour
1 tablespoon baking soda
1 teaspoon salt
Egg substitute equivalent
to 4 eggs, beaten

1 cup vegetable oil
1 quart buttermilk
1 teaspoon vanilla extract
1 (15-ounce) package
raisin bran cereal

Combine the sugar, flour, baking soda and salt in a large bowl and mix well. Add the egg substitute, oil, buttermilk and vanilla and mix well. Stir in the cereal. Cover and store in the refrigerator until baking time.

Fill paper-lined muffin cups with batter. Bake at 400 degrees for 17 to 20 minutes or until the muffins test done.

Yield: 4 to 5 dozen

From the Heart...

"Everyone can be great, because anyone can serve. You don't have to have a college degree to serve. You don't even have to make your subject and verb agree to serve . . . you only need a heart full of grace. A soul generated by love."
—Martin Luther King, Jr.

...of Our House

Banana Buttermilk Buckwheat Pancakes

1 cup all-purpose flour
1/2 cup whole wheat flour
1/2 cup buckwheat flour
2 tablespoons sugar
1 teaspoon salt
1 teaspoon baking soda

4 teaspoons baking powder
2 eggs, lightly beaten
1/4 cup melted butter
1 1/2 cups buttermilk
1/2 cup milk
2 bananas, mashed

Combine the all-purpose flour, whole wheat flour, buckwheat flour, sugar, salt, baking soda and baking powder in a large bowl and mix well.

Combine the eggs, butter, buttermilk, milk and bananas in a medium bowl and mix well. Add to the flour mixture and mix well. Drop by 1/3 cupfuls onto a 350-degree griddle. Cook until lightly browned on both sides.

Yield: 4 to 6 servings

Crepes Stuffed with Ricotta Cheese and Prosciutto

1 (15-ounce) container ricotta cheese
2 ounces finely chopped
prosciutto or ham
1/8 teaspoon salt, or to taste
1 to 2 tablespoons milk
4 eggs, beaten

1/8 teaspoon salt, or to taste
1/4 cup flour
7 tablespoons milk
3 tablespoons melted butter
Grated Parmesan or Romano cheese

For the filling, combine the ricotta cheese and prosciutto in a bowl and mix well. Add 1/8 teaspoon salt and enough of the 1 to 2 tablespoons milk to make of a creamy consistency.

For the crepes, beat the eggs with 1/8 teaspoon salt in a small bowl. Place the flour in a large bowl. Stir in 7 tablespoons milk gradually until smooth. Add the egg mixture gradually, beating constantly. Stir in the melted butter.

Prepare 1 crepe at a time. Melt a small amount of additional butter in a 6-inch skillet. Add 5 or 6 tablespoons of the batter to the skillet, tilting the skillet back and forth so that the batter spreads evenly. Cook slowly until 1 side is set. Turn and cook until the other side is set. Slide the crepe off the skillet onto a board. Repeat the process until all the batter is used.

Place a small amount of filling in the center of each crepe. Overlap the sides of the crepes so that they hold in the filling. Arrange in a single layer in a baking pan or baking dish. Dot each crepe with butter and sprinkle with cheese. Bake at 350 degrees for 15 minutes. Serve hot.

Yield: 4 to 6 servings

Biscotti

2³/4 cups slivered almonds
2 cups flour
1/8 teaspoon salt, or to taste
2 teaspoons baking powder
1 cup sugar

3 eggs
1 1/2 teaspoons vanilla extract
1/2 teaspoon almond extract
1/4 cup vegetable oil

Spread the almonds on a baking sheet and place in a cold oven. Set the oven temperature at 400 degrees. Bake for 9 minutes or until toasted.

Mix the flour, salt and baking powder in a large bowl. Whisk the sugar, eggs, flavorings and oil in a medium bowl. Add to the flour mixture and mix well.

Working with greased hands, divide the batter into halves. Shape into 2 slightly flattened loaves on a buttered and floured cookie sheet.

Bake at 400 degrees for 25 minutes. Remove from the oven. Cool for 10 minutes before cutting into 1/2-inch slices. Stand each slice on its side on the cookie sheet. Bake for 10 minutes longer.

Editor's Note: You may add 1/2 to 1 cup miniature chocolate chips to the batter.

Yield: 3 dozen

Company Eggs

1/2 cup shredded Gruyère or
Swiss cheese
1/4 cup butter
1 cup light cream or whipping cream

1/2 teaspoon salt
1/8 teaspoon pepper, or to taste
1 1/2 teaspoons dry mustard
12 eggs, lightly beaten

Spread the cheese in a buttered 9x13-inch baking dish. Dot with butter. Mix the cream, salt, pepper and mustard in a bowl. Layer half the cream mixture, all the eggs and remaining cream mixture over the cheese in the baking dish. Bake at 325 degrees for 35 minutes or until a knife inserted near the center comes out clean.

Yield: 8 to 10 servings

Eggs Rustica

8 ounces bacon, crisp-cooked,
crumbled
2/3 cup chopped scallions
2 cups shredded Cheddar cheese
12 ounces fresh mushrooms, sliced

Butter
12 eggs
1 1/2 cups whipping cream
1/2 teaspoon salt
1/8 teaspoon pepper

Spread the bacon, scallions and cheese in an 8x10-inch or 9x13-inch baking pan. Sauté the mushrooms in a small amount of butter in a skillet; drain well. Spoon the mushrooms over the cheese in the baking pan. Beat the eggs lightly in a large mixer bowl. Beat in the whipping cream, salt and pepper. Spoon gently over the mushrooms. Bake at 350 degrees for 30 to 35 minutes or until puffed and golden brown. Cut into squares to serve. Garnish with parsley sprigs.

Yield: 8 to 10 servings

Spinach Frittata

3 tablespoons olive oil
1/2 cup thinly sliced onion
10 eggs
1 cup finely chopped spinach
1/3 cup grated Parmesan cheese

1 tablespoon chopped parsley
1 small clove of garlic, crushed
1 teaspoon salt
1/4 teaspoon pepper

Heat the olive oil in a heavy 10-inch ovenproof skillet. Add the onion. Sauté for 5 minutes or until the onion is tender and golden brown.

Combine the eggs, spinach, cheese, parsley, garlic, salt and pepper in a large bowl and whisk well. Spoon into the skillet with the onion. Cook over low heat for 3 minutes or until set, lifting the egg mixture from the bottom with a spatula.

Bake at 350 degrees for 10 minutes or until the top is set. Loosen from the bottom and edge of the skillet with a spatula. Slide onto a serving platter. Cut into wedges to serve.

Yield: 4 to 6 servings

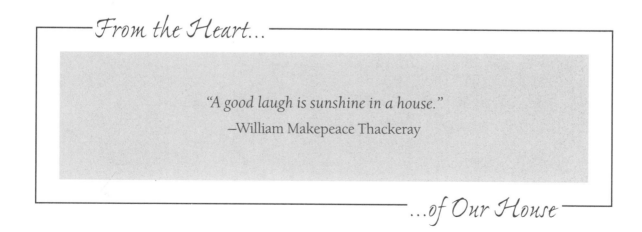

From the Heart...

"A good laugh is sunshine in a house."
—William Makepeace Thackeray

...of Our House

Sherried Crab Quiche

1 recipe (1-crust) pie pastry
1 tablespoon butter, softened
2 cups whipping cream
4 eggs
1 teaspoon salt
4 ounces Swiss cheese, shredded

3 tablespoons butter
2 tablespoons minced onion
2 (6-ounce) packages frozen
snow crab, thawed, drained
2 tablespoons dry sherry
1/8 teaspoon cayenne

Fit the pie pastry into a pie plate. Spread with 1 tablespoon butter and set aside. Whisk the whipping cream, eggs and salt in a medium bowl. Stir in the cheese.

Melt 3 tablespoons butter in a skillet over medium heat. Add the onion. Sauté briefly. Add the onion, crab meat, sherry and cayenne to the egg mixture and mix gently. Spoon into the pie plate.

Bake at 425 degrees for 25 minutes. Reduce the oven temperature to 325 degrees. Bake for 35 minutes or until a knife inserted near the center comes out clean.

Yield: 8 servings

From the Heart...

"Home is not where you live but where they understand you."
—Christian Morgenstern

...of Our House

Creamed Lobster and Johnnycakes

1/4 cup butter
1 teaspoon minced shallots
1/4 cup flour
1 cup fish stock or clam juice
1/4 cup madeira
1 cup whipping cream
1/8 teaspoon nutmeg

1/8 teaspoon salt
1/8 teaspoon freshly ground
black pepper
1/8 teaspoon cayenne
2 cups cooked lobster meat
12 johnnycakes

Melt the butter in a heavy saucepan. Add the shallots. Sauté over medium heat until tender. Stir in the flour. Cook for 2 minutes, stirring constantly; do not brown. Remove from the heat. Whisk until smooth and thick.

Stir in the fish stock and madeira. Stir in the whipping cream. Season with nutmeg, salt, black pepper and cayenne. Fold in the lobster meat. Serve the lobster over stacks of 3 Johnnycakes. Garnish with lobster claw meat.

Yield: 4 servings

Johnnycakes

2 cups white cornmeal
1 1/2 teaspoons salt
2 teaspoons sugar
2 cups boiling water

1/2 cup hot scalded milk
1 egg, lightly beaten
1/2 cup bacon drippings or
vegetable oil

Mix the cornmeal, salt and sugar in a bowl. Add the boiling water and milk and mix well. Stir in the egg. Heat the drippings on a medium-hot griddle or in a heavy skillet. Drop the cornmeal mixture by tablespoonfuls onto the griddle or into the skillet. Fry for 5 minutes per side.

Shrimp with Creamy Dill Sauce

1 pound (25 to 30) cooked peeled
deveined shrimp

Creamy Dill Sauce
Bibb lettuce

Stir the shrimp into the Creamy Dill Sauce in a bowl. Chill, covered, until serving time. Serve on individual lettuce-lined plates or in a lettuce-lined bowl.

Yield: 4 to 6 servings

Creamy Dill Sauce

$\frac{1}{2}$ cup sour cream
$\frac{1}{2}$ cup mayonnaise
$\frac{1}{2}$ cup chopped seeded
peeled cucumber
$\frac{1}{3}$ cup minced onion
$1\frac{1}{2}$ tablespoons chopped dillweed

$1\frac{1}{2}$ teaspoons lemon juice
8 drops of Tabasco sauce
$\frac{1}{4}$ teaspoon caraway seeds
Minced garlic to taste
Salt and pepper to taste

Combine the sour cream, mayonnaise, cucumber, onion, dillweed, lemon juice, Tabasco sauce and caraway seeds in a bowl and mix well. Season with garlic, salt and pepper.

Tomato Mozzarella Tart

3/4 cup plus 2 tablespoons flour
1/4 teaspoon sugar
1/4 teaspoon salt
6 tablespoons unsalted butter,
cut into slices
4 teaspoons ice water
1 tablespoon Dijon mustard

1/2 cup ricotta cheese
4 ounces mozzarella cheese, shredded
3 large tomatoes, thinly sliced
1 clove of garlic, minced
1 teaspoon dried oregano
1/8 teaspoon pepper
2 tablespoons chopped fresh basil

For the pastry, combine the flour, sugar and salt in a food processor fitted with a steel blade. Process in short bursts until mixed. Add the butter 1 slice at a time, processing until the mixture is crumbly and all the butter is incorporated. Add the ice water, mixing for 30 seconds or until the dough forms a ball. Chill, covered, for 1 hour or until firm.

Roll the dough into a 10-inch circle on a floured surface. Fit into a tart pan or pie plate. If using a pie plate, crimp the edge of the pastry halfway up the side. Cover the pastry with foil and line with pie weights. Bake at 325 degrees for 10 minutes. Remove from the oven. Remove the pie weights and foil. Increase the oven temperature to 400 degrees.

Spread the crust with the Dijon mustard, then with the ricotta cheese. Sprinkle with the mozzarella cheese. Arrange the tomato slices in a circular pattern over the cheese. Sprinkle with the garlic, oregano and pepper.

Bake for 45 minutes. Remove from the oven and sprinkle immediately with the basil. Serve hot or at room temperature.

Yield: 5 servings

Soups & Salads

"Volunteering on weekends became a little bit more as time went on, month after month. It also became a way for me to volunteer with my family. I bring my five-year-old and my two-year-old, and my five-year-old has his jobs around the House, too. Hopefully, it will teach them the importance of giving something back to the community."

—Mary Beth Quinn, volunteer

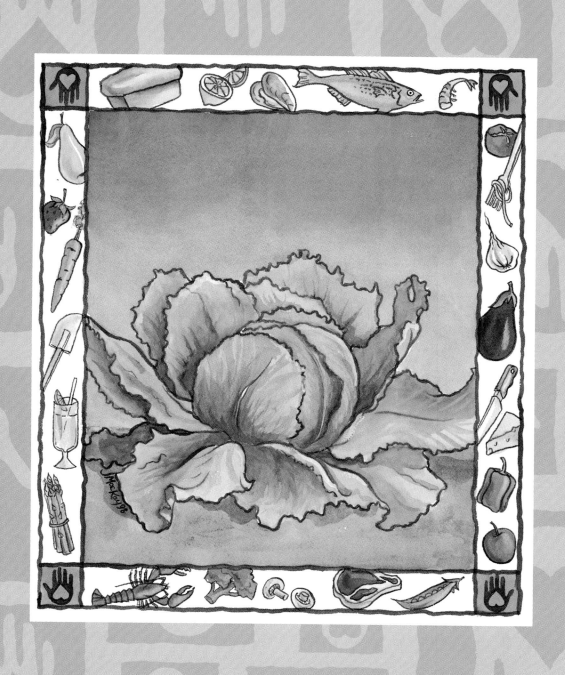

Soups & Salads

Cream of Artichoke Soup 49

Asparagus Soup 50

New England Cheddar Cheese Soup 51

Purée of Butternut Squash and Apple Soup 52

Farmer's Fresh Tomato Soup 53

Nirope Vegetable Soup 54

White Chili 55

Texas Chili 56

Summertime Coleslaw 57

Carrot Raisin Salad 58

Lentil Salad 58

Spinach and Cabbage Salad with Pecans 59

Pasta Salad with Red Wine Vinaigrette 60

Roast Beef Salad with Pesto Vinaigrette 61

Shrimp and Rice Salad 62

Raspberry Vinaigrette 63

Italian Salad Dressing 63

Cream of Artichoke Soup

½ onion, chopped
2 carrots, sliced
2 ribs celery, chopped
¼ cup margarine
1 (4-ounce) can mushrooms,
drained, sliced
1 bay leaf
½ teaspoon thyme
½ teaspoon oregano

⅛ teaspoon cayenne
1 (14-ounce) can artichoke hearts in
water, drained, chopped
4 cups low-sodium chicken broth
¼ cup margarine
3 tablespoons flour
1 cup light cream
Salt and black pepper to taste

Sauté the onion, carrots and celery in ¼ cup margarine in a large saucepan until tender. Add the mushrooms, bay leaf, thyme, oregano, cayenne, artichoke hearts and chicken broth and mix well. Simmer for 15 to 20 minutes or until heated through.

Melt ¼ cup margarine in a small saucepan. Stir in the flour. Cook until thickened, stirring constantly. Stir in the flour mixture. Cook until slightly thickened. Add the cream gradually, stirring constantly. Season with salt and black pepper. Remove and discard bay leaf before serving. Recipe may be doubled.

Yield: 3 to 4 servings

Asparagus Soup

Chef Nancy Verde Barr notes that this "absolutely delicious Calabrian recipe can be prepared with no effort and little time."

2 tablespoons extra-virgin olive oil
2 cloves of garlic, minced
2 pounds asparagus, trimmed, peeled,
cut into 1-inch pieces
Salt and pepper to taste

1 quart chicken broth
4 eggs
1/2 cup freshly grated Parmesan or
Pecorino cheese
6 slices Italian bread, toasted

Heat the olive oil in a stockpot. Add the garlic. Cook until the garlic is golden brown. Add the asparagus to the garlic in the stockpot. Cook until the asparagus begins to change color. Season with salt and pepper.

Add the chicken broth. Bring to a boil; reduce the heat. Simmer for 15 minutes or until the asparagus is tender. Reduce the heat so that the soup is no longer simmering.

Beat the eggs and cheese in a bowl. Ladle a small amount of the hot soup at a time into the egg mixture, stirring constantly. Continue until about 2 cups of soup have been added to the eggs. Stir the egg mixture into the soup in the stockpot gradually. Do not allow the soup to boil or the eggs will scramble. Cook until thickened, stirring frequently.

To serve, place 1 slice of toast in each of 6 soup plates. Ladle soup over the toast. Serve with additional cheese.

Editor's Note: To trim asparagus easily, hold the tip in 1 hand and the base of the stalk in the other. Bend gently. The asparagus will snap, leaving the tender part with the tip.

Yield: 6 servings

New England Cheddar Cheese Soup

½ cup butter
½ cup finely chopped carrot
½ cup finely chopped celery
½ cup finely chopped
green bell pepper
½ cup finely chopped
red bell pepper

½ cup finely chopped onion
1 teaspoon paprika
¾ cup flour
1 quart chicken stock
1 quart hot skim milk
1 pound Cheddar cheese, shredded

Melt the butter in a large saucepan. Add the carrot, celery, green pepper, red pepper and onion. Sauté for 10 minutes. Add the paprika and flour and mix well. Cook for 5 minutes.

Add the chicken stock and mix well. Simmer for 20 minutes. Add the milk. Cook until heated through. Remove from the heat. Add the cheese to the soup, stirring until the cheese is melted. Serve immediately.

Yield: 10 servings

From the Heart...

"The ornament of a house is the friends who frequent it."
—Ralph Waldo Emerson

...of Our House

Purée of Butternut Squash and Apple Soup

Significantly rich in vitamin A, delectable in flavor, and easily stored for months in a cool place, butternut tops the list of winter squash varieties. Avoid purchasing squash that have watery spots, which indicate decay.

5 cups chicken stock
5 cups chopped peeled
butternut squash
1 tablespoon minced onion
1 tablespoon minced celery
1 cup plain nonfat yogurt

1 cup shredded peeled
Granny Smith apple
1 teaspoon sugar
1/4 teaspoon nutmeg
1/4 teaspoon cinnamon

Bring the chicken stock to a boil in a stockpot. Add the squash, onion and celery. Simmer for 30 to 40 minutes or until the squash is tender. Drain well, reserving the broth. Purée the squash mixture in a food processor. Add to the reserved broth in the stockpot. Bring to a boil; remove from the heat. Stir in the yogurt, apple, sugar, nutmeg and cinnamon. Ladle into heated soup bowls. Serve immediately.

Yield: 4 servings

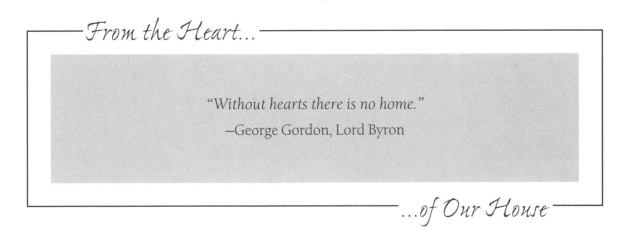

— *From the Heart...*

"Without hearts there is no home."
—George Gordon, Lord Byron

...of Our House

Farmer's Fresh Tomato Soup

Chef Nancy Verde Barr says, "In Italy and later in America, fall was alive with the bustle of whole families harvesting and putting up tomatoes. This Italian farmer's soup is one delicious way of making use of a bumper crop. Tomatoes in Italy were sweeter than the ones the immigrants could grow in New England. I know many Italian-Americans who always add a pinch of sugar to tomato recipes. As with all tomato recipes, the cook really has to be the judge as to whether or not the tomatoes are sweet enough. It's really a matter of balancing the natural acidity in the tomato. The soup should by no means be sweet in terms of sugary."

1/4 cup extra-virgin olive oil
2 medium onions, coarsely chopped
3 cloves of garlic, minced
2 ribs celery, coarsely chopped
3 pounds plum tomatoes, coarsely chopped
Salt to taste
1/8 teaspoon sugar, or to taste

3 slices day-old Italian bread, crusts removed
4 cups hot meat broth
1/2 cup basil leaves, torn into strips
2 tablespoons chopped fresh parsley
2 tablespoons chopped fresh marjoram
2 tablespoons extra-virgin olive oil

Heat 1/4 cup olive oil in a stockpot over medium-low heat. Add the onions, garlic and celery. Cook for 20 minutes or until the garlic is golden brown, stirring occasionally. Add the tomatoes, salt and sugar. Cook, partially covered, for 20 minutes or until the tomatoes are tender.

Place the bread in a small bowl. Add 1 cup of the hot broth to soften. Mash well with a wooden spoon. Add the softened bread and remaining 3 cups broth to the tomatoes, stirring until the bread is completely disintegrated. Simmer for 25 minutes. Add the basil, parsley and marjoram. Simmer for 5 minutes longer.

Purée the soup in a food processor. Return the soup to the stockpot. Adjust the seasonings. Simmer for 10 minutes. Ladle into heated soup bowls. Pour 1 teaspoon olive oil over each serving. Garnish each with 1 sprig of fresh marjoram.

Yield: 6 servings

Nirope Vegetable Soup

1 pound lean ground beef
4 quarts water
1 (28-ounce) can ground
 peeled tomatoes
1/3 cup beef soup base, or
 12 beef bouillon cubes

1 (20-ounce) package frozen
 mixed vegetables
1 teaspoon dried minced onion
1 quart water
1 1/2 cups alphabet macaroni
Salt and pepper to taste

Brown the ground beef in a skillet, stirring until crumbly; drain well. Combine 4 quarts water, tomatoes and soup base in an 8-quart stockpot and mix well. Add the mixed vegetables, ground beef and onion and mix well. Cover and bring to a boil; reduce the heat. Simmer for 1 1/2 hours or until the vegetables are tender, stirring occasionally.

Bring 1 quart water to a boil in a saucepan. Add the macaroni. Cook until tender. Drain and rinse in cold water.

Add the macaroni to the soup and mix well. Season with salt and pepper. Simmer for 15 minutes. Serve hot with crackers. Cooled soup may be frozen in plastic containers.

Yield: 12 to 15 servings

White Chili

1 pound white beans
6 cups (or more) chicken broth
2 cloves of garlic, minced
2 medium onions, chopped
1 tablespoon vegetable oil
2 (4-ounce) cans chopped mild
green chiles, drained
1 1/2 teaspoons oregano

1 teaspoon ground cumin
1/4 teaspoon ground cloves
1/4 teaspoon cayenne
4 cups chopped cooked chicken
Sour cream
Salsa
2 cups shredded Monterey Jack cheese

Soak the beans in water to cover overnight; drain well. Combine the beans, chicken broth, garlic and half the onions in a large stockpot. Bring to a boil; reduce the heat. Simmer for 3 hours or until the beans are tender, adding additional broth if needed.

Sauté the remaining onions in the oil in a skillet. Add the green chiles, oregano, cumin, cloves and cayenne and mix well. Add the chile mixture and chicken to the bean mixture and mix well. Simmer for 1 hour. Ladle into soup bowls. Top each serving with sour cream, salsa and cheese.

Yield: 8 to 10 servings

Texas Chili

True Texas chili does not contain any beans!

4 ounces bacon, chopped
2 pounds beef chuck roast, cut into
1/8-inch cubes
3 yellow onions, chopped
6 cloves of garlic, finely chopped
6 jalapeños, seeded, chopped

1 (28-ounce) can crushed tomatoes
1/4 cup hot or mild chili powder
1 tablespoon cumin seeds
2 teaspoons salt
1 tablespoon oregano

Sauté the bacon in a heated 6-quart stockpot until translucent. Add the beef cubes, onions, garlic and jalapeños. Cook over high heat until the beef is browned and the onions are translucent, stirring frequently to prevent sticking.

Add the tomatoes, chili powder, cumin seeds, salt and oregano to the chili and mix well. Simmer for 1 hour.

Yield: 4 to 6 servings

From the Heart...

"Home is not just a place to sleep, home is where we house our souls."
—Alexandra Stoddard

...of Our House

Summertime Coleslaw

This fruity salad is a new twist to an old-time favorite. Adding fresh raspberries to the salad lightens the flavor and makes it a refreshing accompaniment to all your picnic dishes. And it's naturally low in fat.

2 cups fresh savoy cabbage,
cut into thin strips
1 cup fresh purple cabbage,
cut into thin strips
1 cup shredded peeled carrots
1 1/2 tablespoons finely chopped
red onion

3/4 cup Raspberry Vinaigrette
(page 63)
1/2 cup low-fat or nonfat sour cream
1 tablespoon poppy seeds
2 tablespoons sugar
Salt and pepper to taste
1/2 cup fresh raspberries

Combine all the cabbage, carrots and onion in a large bowl and mix well. Combine the Raspberry Vinaigrette, sour cream, poppy seeds and sugar in a small bowl and mix well. Season with salt and pepper. Add the vinaigrette mixture to the vegetables and toss to mix. Chill, covered, overnight.

Fold the raspberries into the coleslaw just before serving time. Serve in a salad bowl garnished with assorted salad greens.

Yield: 4 servings

Carrot Raisin Salad

½ cup plain nonfat yogurt
2 tablespoons reduced-
calorie mayonnaise
1 teaspoon sugar (optional)
1 pound carrots, peeled, grated

½ cup canned crushed pineapple in
pineapple juice
2 tablespoons raisins
2 teaspoons shredded coconut

Beat the yogurt, mayonnaise and sugar in a large bowl until blended. Add the carrots, pineapple and raisins and toss to coat. Chill, covered, until serving time. Toss again. Sprinkle with the coconut.

Yield: 6 servings

Lentil Salad

1 medium red onion, chopped
8 cloves of garlic, minced,
or to taste
Chopped parsley
Chopped red bell pepper (optional)

Chopped celery (optional)
½ cup balsamic vinegar
½ cup olive oil
1 pound lentils

Mix the onion, garlic, parsley, red pepper, celery, vinegar and olive oil in a bowl. Sort and rinse the lentils. Cook the lentils in boiling water to cover in a saucepan for 15 to 20 minutes or just until firm; do not overcook. Drain well and rinse with cold water. Add the lentils to the parsley mixture and mix gently.

Yield: 4 to 6 servings

Spinach and Cabbage Salad with Pecans

1/3 cup coarsely chopped pecans
10 ounces spinach, torn into
bite-size pieces
1/4 small head red cabbage,
thinly sliced
1/2 small red onion, thinly sliced

1 1/2 tablespoons red wine vinegar
1/2 teaspoon grainy mustard
3 tablespoons extra-virgin olive oil
3 tablespoons buttermilk
Salt and freshly ground pepper to taste

Spread the pecans in a baking pan. Bake at 400 degrees for 8 minutes or until toasted, stirring once. Let cool.

Toss the spinach, cabbage and onion in a large bowl. Chill, covered, until serving time. Whisk the vinegar and mustard in a small bowl. Whisk in the oil, then the buttermilk. Season with salt and pepper. Add the pecans and dressing to the salad just before serving time, tossing to mix.

Yield: 4 servings

From the Heart...

"Shut the door. Not that it lets in the cold but that it lets out the coziness."
–Mark Twain

...of Our House

Pasta Salad with Red Wine Vinaigrette

1 (8-ounce) package small to
medium pasta
1/2 cup julienned red onion
1 cup blanched green beans
1/2 cup blanched finely chopped
Red Bliss potatoes

1 teaspoon drained chopped capers
1/2 cup julienned red bell pepper
1/2 cup julienned yellow bell pepper
Red Wine Vinaigrette

Cook the pasta using the package directions. Drain and rinse under cold water; drain again. Combine the pasta, onion, green beans, potatoes, capers, red pepper and yellow pepper in a large bowl and mix well. Add Red Wine Vinaigrette to the salad and toss well. Garnish with baby greens, Casablanca olives and red pear tomatoes.

Yield: 6 servings

Red Wine Vinaigrette

1/2 cup extra-virgin olive oil
2 cloves of garlic, minced
2 tablespoons red wine vinegar

1 teaspoon fresh lemon juice
1 ounce fresh parsley, chopped
Salt and freshly ground pepper to taste

Whisk the olive oil, garlic, vinegar, lemon juice and parsley in a bowl. Season with salt and pepper.

Roast Beef Salad with Pesto Vinaigrette

2 tablespoons pine nuts
2 heads Boston lettuce, cored,
rinsed, drained
8 radicchio leaves, rinsed, dried

1 pound rare roast beef, cut into
thin strips
Pesto Vinaigrette

Spread the pine nuts in a pie plate. Bake at 300 degrees for 8 to 10 minutes or until toasted, stirring occasionally; set aside. Tear the lettuce into bite-size pieces; shred the radicchio. Line a serving platter or 4 individual plates with the greens. Top with roast beef. Sprinkle with pine nuts. Drizzle with Pesto Vinaigrette.

Yield: 4 servings

Pesto Vinaigrette

$^1/_2$ cup olive oil
1 clove of garlic
1 to 2 cups fresh basil
2 tablespoons pine nuts

1 cup freshly grated Parmesan cheese
$^3/_4$ teaspoon salt
$^1/_4$ cup red wine vinegar
$^1/_4$ cup water

Process the olive oil and garlic in a food processor until the garlic is finely chopped. Add the basil, pine nuts, cheese and salt. Process until fairly smooth. Stir in the vinegar and water.

Shrimp and Rice Salad

6 cups cooked rice
12 ounces shrimp, cooked, chopped
1 cup sliced mushrooms
1 cup slightly blanched pea pods
Chopped pimento (optional)
1 (6-ounce) jar marinated artichoke
hearts, drained, chopped

1 cup sliced green bell pepper
1 cup chopped red onion
1/4 to 1/2 cup raisins
Herbal Vinaigrette

Combine the rice, shrimp, mushrooms, pea pods, pimento, artichoke hearts, green pepper, onion and raisins in a bowl and mix well. Toss with Herbal Vinaigrette. Chill, covered, for 4 to 6 hours.

Yield: 6 to 8 servings

Herbal Vinaigrette

3/4 cup corn oil
3 tablespoons wine vinegar
1 to 2 teaspoons minced garlic
1/4 teaspoon oregano

1/4 teaspoon basil
1 tablespoon lemon juice
Salt and pepper to taste

Combine the corn oil, vinegar, garlic, oregano, basil and lemon juice in a jar with a tight-fitting lid and shake to mix well. Season with salt and pepper.

Raspberry Vinaigrette

2 cups low-sodium chicken stock or
chicken broth, skimmed
1 cup raspberry vinegar
1/4 cup olive oil
2 tablespoons cornstarch

1 tablespoon water
2 tablespoons chopped fresh herbs, or
1 teaspoon dried
1 tablespoon minced garlic
1 1/2 teaspoons sugar

Combine the chicken stock, vinegar and olive oil in a small saucepan. Cook over medium heat until heated through. Whisk in a mixture of the cornstarch and water gradually. Reduce the heat to low. Simmer for 5 minutes, stirring constantly. Remove from the heat and let cool. Stir in the herbs, garlic and sugar. Chill, covered, until serving time.

Yield: 3 1/2 cups

Italian Salad Dressing

1 tablespoon chopped fresh basil
1 tablespoon chopped fresh oregano
1 to 2 cloves of garlic, ends removed
1 tablespoon chopped white onion
1/2 cup balsamic vinegar or
red wine vinegar

1/2 cup water
2 tablespoons freshly grated
Parmesan cheese
1/2 cup canola oil
Salt and freshly ground pepper to taste

Combine the basil, oregano, garlic, onion, vinegar, water and cheese in a food processor container. Purée for 2 minutes. Add the oil in a steady stream with the food processor running. Season with salt and pepper. Store in the refrigerator in a jar with a tight-fitting lid.

Yield: 1 1/2 cups

Rhode Island Specialties: Pasta & Seafood

"I never needed anybody to help me before, but I did when I stayed here.

I was amazed; everyone just welcomes you. They make you feel like this will be

your home for as long as you need it."

—Linda Noonan, parent

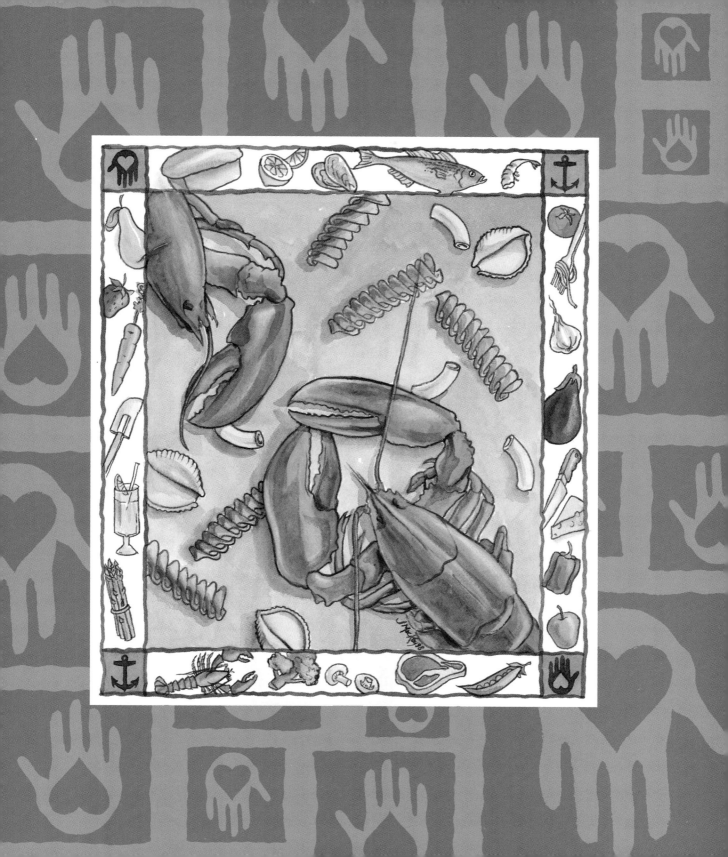

$\mathcal{R}$hode Island Specialties: Pasta & Seafood

Linguini in White Clam Sauce 67

Linguini a la Nirope 68

Macaroni and Cheese for Grownups 69

Orecchiette with Cauliflower, Potatoes
and Kidney Beans 70

Perciatelli with Greens and Seasoned
Bread Crumbs 71

Pasta Providence 72

Creamy Spinach and Tortellini 73

Vermicelli with Lemony
Green Vegetables 74

Pasta Carbonara 75

Due Fettuccini with Prosciutto 76

Baked Ditali with Sweet and
Hot Italian Sausages 77

Baked Ziti with Spinach and Tomatoes 78

Chicken with Penne 79

Penne, Pepper and Salmon in
Garlic Sauce 80

Cardi's Clams and Spaghetti 81

Scampi Fettuccini with Garlic and
Olive Oil 82

Grilled Salmon 83

Salmon with Dijon Sauce 84

Cajun Cod 85

Scrod Imperial 86

Easy Lobster Newburg 87

Venus de Milo Lobster Casserole 88

Seared Scallops with Wild Mushrooms 89

Scallops Nantucket 90

Teriyaki Shrimp 91

Stir-Fried Shrimp with Ginger and Garlic 92

Grilled Shrimp with Prosciutto and Basil 93

Tangy Seafood Kabobs 94

Shrimp with Feta Cheese 95

Creamy Basil Sauce 96

Pesto 96

Mayor Vincent A. Cianci, Jr.'s
Marinara Sauce 97

Sun-Dried Tomato Sauce 97

Linguini in White Clam Sauce

1/2 cup margarine or butter
1/4 cup vegetable oil
3 cloves of garlic, minced
6 ounces sliced mushrooms
1/2 medium onion, chopped
1 cup clam juice

2 tablespoons parsley
2 cans whole baby clams
3/4 cup white wine
1 (16-ounce) package linguini
Freshly grated Parmesan cheese

Heat the margarine and oil in a large skillet over low heat. Add the garlic, mushrooms and onion. Cook until the garlic is golden brown, stirring constantly.

Add the clam juice and parsley to the garlic mixture. Simmer for 10 minutes. Add the clams and wine. Simmer for 10 minutes, stirring constantly.

Cook the linguini using the package directions; drain well. Serve the clam sauce over the linguini. Sprinkle with Parmesan cheese. May substitute chopped fresh clams for the canned clams.

Yield: 4 servings

From the Heart...

"The ache for home lives in all of us, the safe place where we can go as we are and not be questioned."
—Maya Angelou

...of Our House

Linguini à la Nirope

1 tablespoon chopped garlic
1/4 cup olive oil
1 pound (15 to 20) large shrimp
3 small zucchini, cut into 1/2-inch slices
3 small yellow summer squash,
cut into 1/2-inch slices
1 large red bell pepper, chopped

3 carrots, peeled, cut diagonally into
thin slices
2 teaspoons garlic salt
pepper to taste
2 quarts water
1 pound linguini
1/4 cup olive oil

Sauté the garlic in 1/4 cup olive oil in a large skillet. Add the shrimp. Sauté until the shrimp turn pink. Add the zucchini, squash, bell pepper and carrots to the shrimp mixture. Cook, covered, for 3 to 5 minutes or just until tender; do not overcook. Season with garlic salt and pepper.

Bring the water to a boil in a stockpot. Add the linguini. Cook until al dente; drain and rinse. Toss the linguini with 1/4 cup olive oil. Place in a pasta dish. Spoon the shrimp mixture over the top.

Yield: 4 servings

From the Heart...

*"A home is not home unless it contains food and fire for
the mind as well as for the body."*
—Sarah Margaret Fuller

...of Our House

Macaroni and Cheese for Grownups

1 pound macaroni	1/2 cup shredded Gruyère cheese
1/4 cup butter	1/2 cup shredded Swiss cheese
3 tablespoons flour	1/2 teaspoon thyme
2 cups chicken stock	1/8 teaspoon nutmeg
1/4 cup sherry	Salt and cayenne to taste
2 cups milk	1/4 cup bread crumbs
1 cup shredded fontina cheese	1/4 cup grated Parmesan cheese

Boil the macaroni in water to cover in a saucepan until slightly undercooked; drain well. Melt the butter in a skillet. Stir in the flour. Cook for 1 minute, stirring constantly. Whisk in the chicken stock gradually. Boil for 2 minutes. Whisk in the sherry and milk. Bring to a boil; remove from the heat.

Add the fontina cheese, Gruyère cheese and Swiss cheese to the chicken stock, stirring constantly until the cheeses are melted. Stir in the macaroni. Season with thyme, nutmeg, salt and cayenne.

Spoon the macaroni mixture into a 9x13-inch baking pan. Sprinkle with the bread crumbs and Parmesan cheese. Bake at 375 degrees for 30 minutes.

Yield: 8 servings

Orecchiette with Cauliflower, Potatoes and Kidney Beans

Florets of 1 medium cauliflower
12 ounces potatoes, peeled, chopped
Salt to taste
1 chicken bouillon cube
1/2 cup olive oil
4 cloves of garlic, finely chopped

1 (16-ounce) can red kidney beans,
drained, rinsed
Black pepper to taste
Crushed red pepper to taste
1 pound orecchiette
3/4 cup grated Romano cheese

Soak the cauliflower in cold water for 30 minutes; drain well. Soak the potatoes in cold water for 30 minutes; drain well.

Bring a large stockpot of cold water to a boil. Add salt and cauliflower. Cook for 4 minutes. Remove the cauliflower with a slotted spoon and set aside. Add the potatoes to the cooking liquid in the stockpot. Cook for 6 minutes. Remove the potatoes with a slotted spoon and set aside. Reserve the cooking liquid.

Combine 1 1/2 cups of the cooking liquid with the bouillon cube in a bowl and mix well. Set aside.

Heat the olive oil in a large heavy skillet. Add the garlic. Sauté just until golden brown. Add the cauliflower, potatoes and beans. Sauté for 3 minutes. Season with salt, black pepper and red pepper. Add the bouillon mixture. Cook for 10 to 15 minutes or until heated through. Cook the orecchiette in the remaining cooking liquid in a stockpot; drain well.

Combine the orecchiette, cauliflower mixture and cheese in a large serving bowl and toss well. Serve immediately.

Yield: 4 to 6 servings

Perciatelli with Greens and Seasoned Bread Crumbs

3 tablespoons olive oil
2 cups fresh French or Italian
bread crumbs
1/2 cup freshly grated
Pecorino Romano cheese
1 tablespoon grated lemon peel
1 tablespoon dried oregano
1 pound perciatelli or spaghetti
3 tablespoons olive oil

4 cloves of garlic, chopped
3 bunches greens, such as kale,
mustard greens and/or
dandelion greens, stems removed,
sliced crosswise
1 tablespoon olive oil
1/2 cup freshly grated
Pecorino Romano cheese
Salt and pepper to taste

Heat 3 tablespoons olive oil in a large heavy skillet over medium-high heat. Add the bread crumbs. Cook for 3 minutes or until crisp and golden brown, stirring constantly. Mix the bread crumbs, 1/2 cup cheese, lemon peel and oregano in a bowl. Let stand, covered, until needed. May be prepared up to 4 hours ahead.

Cook the pasta in a large stockpot of boiling salted water until al dente, stirring occasionally. Heat 3 tablespoons olive oil in a large Dutch oven over medium-high heat. Add the garlic. Cook for 1 minute or until lightly browned, stirring constantly. If using kale, add the kale and cook for 1 minute or until wilted, stirring constantly. Add the mustard greens and/or dandelion greens. Cook for 2 minutes or until wilted, stirring constantly.

Drain the pasta, reserving 1 1/2 cups of the cooking liquid. Return the pasta to the stockpot. Add 1 tablespoon oil, cooked greens and reserved cooking liquid, tossing to coat. Add 1/2 cup cheese. Season generously with salt and pepper. Remove the pasta to a serving bowl. Top with the seasoned bread crumbs.

Yield: 4 servings

Pasta Providence

1 (6-ounce) jar marinated
artichoke hearts
8 ounces sliced mushrooms
1 tablespoon grated onion
1 clove of garlic, minced
2 cups fresh tomato sauce
1 cup dry white wine
1 (2-ounce) can sliced
black olives, drained

2 teaspoons dried basil
2 teaspoons dried oregano
1 teaspoon salt
1/2 teaspoon fennel seeds
1/4 teaspoon freshly ground pepper
1 (16-ounce) package spaghetti or
other thin pasta
Freshly grated Parmesan cheese

Drain and coarsely chop the artichoke hearts, reserving the marinade. Heat the reserved marinade in a large sauté pan over medium heat until bubbly. Add the mushrooms, onion and garlic. Sauté over high heat for 5 minutes.

Add the artichoke hearts, tomato sauce, wine, olives, basil, oregano, salt, fennel seeds and pepper to the mushroom mixture. Simmer for 20 minutes.

Cook the spaghetti using the package directions; drain well. Remove the spaghetti to a serving bowl. Spoon the sauce over the spaghetti. Sprinkle with Parmesan cheese.

Yield: 4 to 6 servings

Creamy Spinach and Tortellini

1 pound fresh or frozen tortellini
2 tablespoons olive oil
1/2 cup chopped onion
3 cloves of garlic, minced
1 (10-ounce) package frozen chopped
spinach, thawed
1 cup chopped tomato

1/4 cup chopped fresh basil
1/2 teaspoon salt
1/2 teaspoon pepper
1 cup whipping cream
1/4 cup grated Parmesan or
Romano cheese

Cook the tortellini in water to cover in a saucepan to desired degree of doneness. Drain and rinse with hot water.

Heat the olive oil in a large skillet over medium heat. Add the onion and garlic. Cook for 4 minutes or until lightly browned. Add the spinach, tomato, basil, salt and pepper. Cook for 5 minutes, stirring occasionally.

Stir the whipping cream and cheese into the spinach mixture. Cook just until boiling; reduce the heat to low. Add the tortellini and mix well. Cook for 4 to 5 minutes or until heated through. Serve with additional Parmesan cheese.

Yield: 4 servings

Vermicelli with Lemony Green Vegetables

1 (7-ounce) package vermicelli
4 cups mixed bite-size
green vegetables, such as asparagus,
broccoli, pea pods, green beans
and/or zucchini
1/4 cup margarine or butter

1 tablespoon grated lemon peel
1/2 cup milk
3 ounces cream cheese, cut into
cubes, softened
1/4 cup grated Parmesan cheese
Coarsely ground pepper

Cook the vermicelli using the package directions. Combine the vegetables and margarine in a 10-inch skillet. Cook over medium heat for 7 minutes or until tender-crisp, stirring frequently. Toss with the lemon peel. Remove the vegetables and keep warm.

Heat the milk and cream cheese in the skillet until the cream cheese is melted, stirring until smooth and creamy. Stir in the Parmesan cheese.

Drain the vermicelli and toss with the cheese sauce. Serve the vegetables over the vermicelli. Sprinkle with pepper. Garnish with lemon wedges.

Yield: 4 servings

Pasta Carbonara

2 tablespoons butter
1 tablespoon olive oil
6 slices pancetta or bacon, cut into
cubes (see Editor's Note)
4 egg yolks

¹/₃ cup whipping cream
¹/₃ cup grated Parmesan cheese
Salt and freshly ground pepper to taste
1 pound linguini or other thin pasta

Heat the butter and olive oil in a skillet. Add the pancetta. Cook until lightly browned. Set aside and keep warm. Beat the egg yolks in a large bowl. Beat in the whipping cream, cheese, salt and pepper.

Cook the linguini in boiling water to cover in a saucepan until al dente; drain in a colander. Add the pasta immediately to the cream mixture and toss quickly. Add the bacon and toss to mix. Serve with additional Parmesan cheese.

Editor's Note: Pancetta is an unsmoked Italian bacon. Smoked bacon should be blanched quickly to reduce its smokiness; drain well before using.

Yield: 4 servings

Due Fettuccini with Prosciutto

8 ounces fettuccini
8 ounces spinach fettuccini
1/2 cup margarine
3/4 cup olive oil
2 (16-ounce) cans artichoke
hearts, drained, chopped

3 cloves of garlic, minced
1 (16-ounce) can sliced
black olives, drained
8 ounces sliced prosciutto
Salt and pepper to taste

Cook all the fettuccini in boiling water to cover in a saucepan until al dente. Melt the margarine in a 10-inch sauté pan or skillet. Add the olive oil, artichoke hearts, garlic, olives and prosciutto. Sauté until heated through.

Drain the fettuccini and place in a serving bowl. Add the prosciutto mixture and toss well. Season with salt and pepper. Serve immediately with grated Parmesan cheese, chianti or merlot, and crusty Italian bread.

Yield: 8 servings

From the Heart...

"To build a house is one thing, but to make it a home is quite another."
—Louis L'Amour

...of Our House

Baked Ditali with Sweet and Hot Italian Sausages

1¹/₂ pounds ditali or other small pasta
1 tablespoon olive oil
1 pound sweet Italian sausage,
  casings removed

1 pound hot Italian sausage,
  casings removed
4 cups tomato sauce
1¹/₂ cups ricotta cheese
1 cup freshly grated Parmesan cheese

Cook the ditali in boiling water to cover in a saucepan until barely chewable; drain well. Heat the olive oil in a saucepan. Add the sausages. Cook until evenly browned. Remove the sausages and slice thinly.

Drain the olive oil from the saucepan, leaving the browned bits in the saucepan. Add the tomato sauce and sausage slices. Simmer, covered, for 20 minutes.

Alternate layers of the ditali, meat sauce, ricotta cheese and Parmesan cheese in a buttered baking dish until all the ingredients are used, ending with layers of sauce and cheese. Bake at 350 degrees for 25 minutes or until the sauce is bubbly.

Yield: 6 to 8 servings

Baked Ziti with Spinach and Tomatoes

12 ounces hot Italian sausage,
casings removed
1 medium onion, chopped
3 large cloves of garlic, chopped
1 (28-ounce) can chopped
peeled tomatoes
1/4 cup pesto

Salt and pepper to taste
10 ounces ziti or penne pasta,
cooked, drained
8 cups spinach leaves
6 ounces mozzarella cheese,
cut into cubes
1 cup grated Parmesan cheese

Heat a large heavy saucepan over medium-high heat. Add the sausage, onion and garlic. Sauté for 10 minutes or until the sausage is cooked through, stirring until the sausage is crumbly. Add the undrained tomatoes. Simmer for 10 minutes or until slightly thickened, stirring occasionally. Stir in the pesto. Season with salt and pepper. May be prepared up to 1 day ahead and stored, covered, in the refrigerator. Return to a simmer before continuing with the recipe.

Combine the ziti, spinach, mozzarella cheese and 1/3 cup of the Parmesan cheese in a large bowl. Stir in the hot tomato sauce. Spoon into a lightly oiled 9x13-inch glass baking dish. Sprinkle with the remaining 2/3 cup Parmesan cheese. Bake for 30 minutes or until the sauce is bubbly and the Parmesan cheese is melted. Serve with a green salad, crusty garlic bread and a light red wine, such as a Beaujolais.

Yield: 4 servings

Chicken with Penne

1 gallon salted water
1 pound penne
3 tablespoons olive oil
1 1/2 pounds boneless chicken breast,
  coarsely chopped
8 ounces chopped ham
6 ounces sliced mushrooms
6 cloves of garlic, finely chopped

4 ounces fresh or frozen shelled peas
1 cup whipping cream
1/2 cup butter
2 tablespoons chopped scallions
3 ounces Parmesan cheese, grated
Salt and pepper to taste
Chopped parsley to taste

Bring the water to a boil in a large stockpot. Add the pasta. Cook until al dente, stirring frequently; drain well.

Heat a large sauté pan until very hot. Add the olive oil and chicken. Cook for 2 minutes or until the chicken is seared. Add the ham, mushrooms and garlic. Sauté for 2 minutes. Add the peas and whipping cream. Cook until reduced by 1/2, stirring frequently. Add the pasta. Stir in the butter, scallions and cheese. Remove the pasta mixture to a serving bowl. Season with salt and pepper. Sprinkle with parsley.

Yield: 4 to 6 servings

$\mathcal{P}$enne, Pepper and Salmon in Garlic Sauce

1 pound penne or other tubular pasta
6 ounces thinly sliced smoked salmon,
cut into 1/3x2-inch strips

1 large red bell pepper, julienned
1 small red onion, thinly sliced
Garlic Sauce

Cook the penne in a large stockpot of boiling salted water until tender; drain well. Remove to a large bowl. Reserve 16 salmon strips for a garnish. Add the remaining salmon strips, red pepper strips and onion to the pasta. Add Garlic Sauce and toss gently. Divide the pasta mixture evenly among 4 plates. Garnish each serving with a sprig of fresh dill and 4 of the reserved salmon strips. Serve warm or at room temperature.

Yield: 4 servings

Garlic Sauce

1/2 cup whipping cream
4 cloves of garlic, lightly crushed
1/4 cup fresh lemon juice
3/4 cup olive oil

2 tablespoons minced fresh dill
2 tablespoons minced fresh parsley
Salt and pepper to taste

Bring the whipping cream to a boil in a saucepan over medium heat. Add the garlic. Simmer for 15 minutes or until the garlic is tender and the whipping cream is reduced to approximately 1/4 cup. Purée the cream mixture in a food processor or blender until very smooth. Add the lemon juice and olive oil. Process until emulsified. Blend in the dill, parsley, salt and pepper.

Cardi's Clams and Spaghetti

1 teaspoon chopped garlic
1 teaspoon dried onion
1/4 cup olive oil
1 (28-ounce) can ground
peeled tomatoes
3 1/2 cups water
2 1/2 cups fresh baby clams with juice,
or 2 (10-ounce) cans baby clams
1/2 teaspoon salt
1/2 teaspoon black pepper

2 tablespoons sugar
1/8 teaspoon red pepper flakes,
or to taste
1/2 cup chopped fresh basil, or
1 tablespoon dried
2 quarts water
1 pound spaghetti
Grated Parmesan or Romano
cheese (optional)

Sauté the garlic and onion in the olive oil in a large saucepan just until browned. Remove from the heat. Add the tomatoes, 3 1/2 cups water, clams, salt, black pepper, sugar, red pepper and basil and mix well. Cook for 25 minutes or until the sauce is slightly thickened, stirring occasionally.

Bring 2 quarts water to a boil in a large stockpot. Add the spaghetti. Cook just until tender; do not overcook. Drain the spaghetti; do not rinse. Place the spaghetti in a large flat pasta dish or bowl. Ladle some of the sauce over the top, tossing to coat. Top with Parmesan cheese. Serve with the remaining sauce.

Yield: 4 servings

Scampi Fettuccini with Garlic and Olive Oil

Shrimp is an excellent and tasty source of protein. In this fettuccini recipe, large shrimp are briefly poached in white wine, then cooked in a sauce that is high in garlic and low in oil. Since it keeps well on a heated tray, this fettuccini is an elegant main dish for a party buffet.

2 quarts water	2 tablespoons olive oil
1 pound fresh fettuccini	2 tablespoons minced garlic
1 pound large shrimp, peeled, deveined	1/4 cup minced red bell pepper
	1/4 cup chopped parsley
1/2 cup dry white wine	1/4 cup grated Parmesan cheese

Bring the water to a boil in a large stockpot over high heat. Add the fettuccini. Cook for 3 minutes; drain well and refresh under cold water.

Sauté the shrimp in white wine in a large skillet over medium-high heat for 4 to 5 minutes or until the shrimp turn pink. Remove the shrimp and set aside.

Drain all but 2 tablespoons wine from the skillet. Add the olive oil, garlic and red pepper to the skillet. Cook over medium-high heat for 5 minutes, stirring frequently. Add the parsley, shrimp and fettuccini. Cook until heated through, stirring frequently. Top with the cheese.

Yield: 4 servings

Grilled Salmon

You can use either of these marinades for Grilled Salmon, or, for a large group, double the marinade recipes and marinate half the salmon in the teriyaki marinade and half in the garlic basil marinade.

1½ pounds salmon fillet

Teriyaki Marinade or
Garlic Basil Marinade

Place the salmon skin side down on a large piece of foil. Fold up the edges of the foil to make a ½-inch rim on all sides. Pour either marinade over the salmon. Marinate for 15 minutes. Place the salmon on the foil on the rack of a medium-hot grill. Grill with the lid closed until the salmon reaches the desired degree of doneness, basting occasionally with the remaining marinade. Salmon may instead be broiled.

Yield: 4 servings

Teriyaki Marinade

½ cup soy sauce
2 cloves of garlic, chopped

1 teaspoon grated fresh gingerroot

Combine the soy sauce, garlic and gingerroot in a medium bowl and mix well.

Garlic Basil Marinade

½ cup olive oil
3 cloves of garlic, chopped

½ cup chopped fresh basil

Combine the olive oil, garlic and basil in a medium bowl and mix well.

Salmon with Dijon Sauce

A favorite French bistro recipe, Salmon with Dijon Sauce can be served cool or hot. It makes a light and elegant luncheon dish. The salmon is lightly poached in wine to retain its tender texture. The flavor of the wine combines well with the piquant mustard and dill of the sauce. The sauce can be prepared ahead and kept for one week in the refrigerator. The sauce is great on sandwiches, too.

4 large salmon steaks	1/4 cup minced shallots
1 cup dry white wine	Dijon Sauce

Place the salmon steaks in a large deep baking pan. Cover with the wine. Sprinkle with the shallots. Bake at 400 degrees for 12 to 15 minutes or until the salmon is the desired degree of doneness, basting frequently with the wine. Serve Dijon Sauce over the salmon.

Yield: 4 servings

Dijon Sauce

3 tablespoons minced fresh dill	1 tablespoon light honey
1/4 cup plain nonfat yogurt	1/4 cup lemon juice
1/4 cup Dijon mustard	

Combine the dill, yogurt, Dijon mustard, honey and lemon juice in a small bowl and mix until smooth.

Cajun Cod

This fish makes a delicious light dinner when served with salad, rice pilaf and French bread.

2 tablespoons plain low-fat yogurt
1 tablespoon lime juice or lemon juice
1 clove of garlic, crushed
1 teaspoon ground cumin
1 teaspoon paprika

1 teaspoon dry mustard
1/2 teaspoon cayenne
1/2 teaspoon dried thyme
1/2 teaspoon dried oregano
4 (6-ounce) cod steaks

Combine the yogurt and lime juice in a small bowl and mix well. Combine the garlic, cumin, paprika, mustard, cayenne, thyme and oregano in a medium bowl and mix well.

Pat the fish dry. Brush lightly with the yogurt mixture. Coat with the mustard mixture. Place the fish in a heavy skillet sprayed with nonstick cooking spray. Cook over high heat for 8 minutes or until browned and cooked through, turning once. May substitute swordfish, tuna or halibut steaks for the cod steaks.

Yield: 4 servings

From the Heart...

"When love adorns a home, other ornaments are secondary."
—Anonymous

...of Our House

Scrod Imperial

1 pound scrod or cod, skin removed
1/2 cup water
1/4 cup bread crumbs
2 teaspoons butter
1/2 cup crab meat

1 tablespoon dry sherry
1 clove of garlic, chopped
2 tablespoons melted butter
1/4 cup chopped parsley

Cut the scrod into 2 pieces. Place skin side down in a casserole. Add the water. Top with the crumbs and 2 teaspoons butter. Bake at 350 degrees for 15 to 20 minutes or until the scrod reaches the desired degree of doneness.

Combine the crab meat, sherry, garlic, melted butter and parsley in a saucepan. Cook over low heat until heated through, stirring occasionally.

Remove the scrod to heated plates with a spatula. Spoon the crab meat mixture over and around the fish. Serve immediately.

Yield: 2 servings

Easy Lobster Newburg

½ cup melted butter or margarine
½ cup flour
1 teaspoon dry mustard
1 teaspoon paprika
1½ cups milk
1 cup whipping cream

2 pounds lobster meat,
cooked, chopped
1 cup sliced mushrooms
2 teaspoons salt
½ cup sherry (optional)

Combine the butter, flour, mustard and paprika in a saucepan. Cook over low heat for 2 to 3 minutes or until heated through, stirring occasionally. Add the milk and whipping cream gradually. Cook until smooth and thickened, stirring constantly.

Stir the lobster meat, mushrooms, salt and sherry into the cream mixture. Remove to a chafing dish set on low heat. Serve over buttered baked rice.

Yield: 8 to 10 servings

From the Heart...

"Those who bring sunshine to the lives of others cannot keep it from themselves."
—James M. Barrie

...of Our House

Venus de Milo Lobster Casserole

1 cup milk
3 tablespoon butter
3 tablespoons flour
1/8 teaspoon salt, or to taste
1/8 teaspoon pepper, or to taste
1 teaspoon dry mustard

1 teaspoon parsley flakes
Chablis to taste
2 pounds lobster meat,
cut into chunks
1 cup crushed butter crackers
1/4 cup melted butter

Bring the milk to a boil in a small saucepan. Simmer until needed. Melt 3 tablespoons butter in a large saucepan. Stir in the flour. Cook for 3 minutes, stirring constantly. Stir in the milk. Cook until thickened, stirring constantly. Add the salt, pepper, mustard and parsley. Add a splash of Chablis. Stir in the lobster meat.

Spoon the lobster mixture into a casserole. Top with a mixture of the butter cracker crumbs and 1/4 cup butter. Bake at 350 degrees for 15 to 20 minutes or until heated through.

Yield: 6 servings

Seared Scallops with Wild Mushrooms

2 tablespoons olive oil	1 tablespoon minced fresh gingerroot
24 large sea scallops	1 tablespoon minced garlic
24 medium oyster mushrooms or	1/4 cup orange liqueur
other mushrooms	2 cups bottled clam juice
1 red bell pepper, julienned	9 cups drained hot cooked linguini
2 tablespoons minced shallots	Salt and pepper to taste

Heat the olive oil in a large skillet over high heat. Add the scallops. Cook for 10 seconds or until seared, stirring constantly. Add the mushrooms, red pepper, shallots, gingerroot and garlic. Cook for 1 minute. Add the liqueur. Cook until the liqueur is hot.

Remove the skillet from the heat. Ignite the liqueur carefully with a match. Return to the heat when the flame has gone out. Add the clam juice. Cook until reduced by 1/3. Toss the scallop mixture with the linguini in a bowl. Season with salt and pepper. Serve immediately.

Yield: 6 servings

Scallops Nantucket

½ cup butter
2 tablespoons sherry or vermouth
1 pound large scallops, drained

1 cup shredded Cheddar cheese
1 cup shredded Monterey Jack cheese
1 cup bread crumbs

Melt the butter in a shallow casserole in a 375-degree oven. Remove the casserole from the oven. Stir in the sherry. Add the scallops, using no more than 2 layers.

Mix the Cheddar cheese and Monterey Jack cheese in a bowl. Sprinkle over the scallops. Top with the bread crumbs. Bake at 375 degrees for 20 minutes or until the cheeses are bubbly and the scallops are cooked through.

Yield: 6 servings

From the Heart...

"All that we send into the lives of others comes back into our own."
–Edwin Markham

...of Our House

Teriyaki Shrimp

You can use the sauce from this recipe for marinating four boneless skinless chicken breasts for 30 minutes to several hours before broiling or grilling. It is also delicious as a marinade for fresh tuna steaks. For a garnish, toast 2 tablespoons sesame seeds in a dry skillet over medium heat for 3 to 5 minutes or until lightly browned.

1 tablespoon grated fresh gingerroot
2 cloves of garlic, minced
2 green onions, chopped
1/4 cup soy sauce
2 tablespoons honey
1 tablespoon rice wine vinegar

1 1/2 teaspoons sesame oil
1 pound (about 24) shrimp,
peeled, deveined
1 tablespoon vegetable oil
1/2 teaspoon cornstarch
1 tablespoon water

Combine the gingerroot, garlic, green onions, soy sauce, honey, vinegar and sesame oil in a large bowl and mix well. Remove and reserve half the marinade. Combine the shrimp with the remaining marinade in a bowl and toss to coat. Marinate, covered, in the refrigerator for 30 minutes to 4 hours.

Remove the shrimp from the marinade, discarding the remaining marinade. Heat the vegetable oil in a wok or large skillet over medium-high heat. Add the shrimp. Sauté for 4 to 5 minutes or until the shrimp turn pink. Remove and keep warm.

Pour the reserved marinade into the skillet. Bring to a boil over medium-high heat. Stir in a mixture of the cornstarch and water. Cook for 1 minute or until thickened, stirring constantly. Add the shrimp, stirring to coat. Spoon the shrimp onto a serving plate. Sprinkle with sesame seeds. Serve with steamed rice.

Yield: 4 servings

Stir-Fried Shrimp with Ginger and Garlic

1/4 cup dry white wine
2 tablespoons soy sauce
1 teaspoon vinegar
1/8 teaspoon sugar, or to taste
1 pound shrimp, peeled, deveined

1 tablespoon minced gingerroot
1 tablespoon minced garlic
2 tablespoons minced green onions
3 tablespoons peanut oil

Mix the wine, soy sauce, vinegar and sugar in a large bowl, stirring until the sugar is dissolved. Add the shrimp, tossing to coat. Marinate for 20 minutes. Mix the gingerroot, garlic and green onions in a small bowl.

Remove the shrimp from the marinade, reserving the remaining marinade. Heat a wok or large skillet over medium-high heat. Add the peanut oil in a thin stream around the skillet, tilting to let the oil run into the center. Add the ginger mixture. Adjust the heat so that the mixture sizzles without burning.

Stir-fry for 30 seconds or until the mixture is very fragrant. Add the shrimp. Stir-fry for 30 seconds or until the shrimp begin to stiffen. Add the marinade. Cook until most of the liquid has evaporated, stirring constantly.

If the shrimp are not quite done, add a few tablespoons of water and cook until the shrimp turn pink and the water has evaporated. The sauce should cling to the shrimp, leaving very little in the wok. Remove to a serving dish. Serve immediately.

Yield: 4 servings

Grilled Shrimp with Prosciutto and Basil

1 cup dry white wine
1 cup olive oil
¼ cup lemon juice
2 cloves of garlic, minced
2 tablespoons Dijon mustard

½ cup chopped fresh basil
Fresh cracked pepper to taste
24 jumbo shrimp
24 large fresh basil leaves
24 thin slices prosciutto

Combine the wine, olive oil, lemon juice, garlic, Dijon mustard, chopped basil and pepper in a bowl and mix well. Peel and devein the shrimp, leaving the tails intact. Place the shrimp in a shallow dish or pan. Add the wine mixture. Marinate, covered, in the refrigerator for 3 hours or longer. Remove the shrimp from the marinade, reserving the remaining marinade. Wrap each shrimp with a basil leaf, then a prosciutto slice. Thread the shrimp onto skewers. Place on a rack on a preheated grill. Grill for several minutes per side or until the shrimp turn pink, basting occasionally with the reserved marinade.

Yield: 4 servings

From the Heart...

"It is the laugh of a baby, the song of a mother, the strength of a father.
Warmth of living hearts, light from happy eyes, kindness, loyalty,
comradeship . . . Where joy is shared and sorrow eased . . . Where even
the teakettle sings from happiness. This is home."
    –Ernestine Schumann-Heink

...of Our House

$\mathcal{T}$angy Seafood Kabobs

1/2 cup beer
1/4 cup soy sauce
1 teaspoon chopped garlic
1/2 teaspoon chopped fresh gingerroot
or ground ginger
2 tablespoons honey
1 tablespoon chopped hot
pepper (optional)
1/4 cup olive oil

2 pounds large prawns, sea scallops
and/or swordfish
16 cherry tomatoes
16 mushrooms
1 red bell pepper, cut into
1-inch pieces
1 green bell pepper, cut into
1-inch pieces

Combine the beer, soy sauce, garlic, gingerroot, honey, hot pepper and olive oil in a shallow dish or pan and mix well. Peel the shrimp, cut the scallops into halves and/or cut the swordfish into 1-inch cubes. Marinate the seafood, covered, in the beer mixture in the refrigerator overnight.

Remove the seafood from the marinade, reserving the remaining marinade. Thread the seafood onto skewers alternately with the cherry tomatoes, mushrooms, red pepper pieces and green pepper pieces.

Grill or broil for 8 to 10 minutes or until the seafood reaches the desired degree of doneness, turning once and basting occasionally with half the reserved marinade.

Serve with rice, orzo or couscous. Heat the remaining half of the marinade in a saucepan and spoon over the rice.

Yield: 4 servings

Shrimp with Feta Cheese

1 tablespoon lemon juice
1¼ pounds medium shrimp,
peeled, deveined
2 tablespoons olive oil
¼ cup chopped onion
½ bunch green onions, chopped
1 clove of garlic, minced

1½ cups canned chopped tomatoes
¼ cup dry white wine
1 tablespoon butter
1 tablespoon ouzo or brandy
¼ teaspoon oregano
1 tablespoon chopped parsley
4 ounces feta cheese, crumbled

Pour the lemon juice over the shrimp in a bowl or shallow dish. Let stand, covered, until needed. Heat the olive oil in a heavy skillet. Add the onion, green onions and garlic. Sauté until the vegetables are tender. Add the tomatoes and wine. Simmer for 15 minutes.

Remove the shrimp from the lemon juice, discarding the remaining lemon juice. Melt the butter in a large skillet. Add the shrimp. Sauté for 3 to 4 minutes or until the shrimp turn pink.

Warm the ouzo in a small saucepan. Remove from the heat and ignite carefully. Pour over the shrimp after the flame has burned out. Add the oregano and parsley. Spoon the shrimp into a 1½-quart casserole, leaving the cooking liquid in the skillet.

Stir the cooking liquid into the tomato sauce. Spoon over the shrimp. Top with the cheese. Bake at 375 degrees for 15 minutes or until bubbly and heated through.

May be prepared ahead and stored in the refrigerator until baking time. Length of baking time may need to be adjusted.

Yield: 8 servings

Creamy Basil Sauce

2 cups skim milk
1 clove of garlic, chopped
1 teaspoon chopped onion
¼ cup skim milk
¼ cup flour

½ bunch fresh basil, stems
removed, rinsed
1 teaspoon grated Parmesan cheese
Salt and pepper to taste

Heat 2 cups skim milk in a medium saucepan over medium heat to just below the boiling point. Add the garlic and onion as the milk heats, pressing down to submerge in the milk. Whisk ¼ cup skim milk and flour in a bowl. Add to the garlic mixture gradually, whisking constantly. Return to a gentle simmer. Cook for 10 minutes, stirring frequently. Remove from the heat. Purée the basil leaves in a food processor or blender. Add the basil and cheese to the milk mixture and mix well. Season with salt and pepper.

Yield: 4 to 6 servings

Pesto

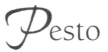

1 clove of garlic, end removed
2 bunches fresh basil, stems
removed, rinsed
½ cup lightly toasted pine nuts

3 to 4 tablespoons freshly grated
Parmesan cheese
2 tablespoons (or more) olive oil
½ teaspoon freshly ground pepper

Combine the garlic, basil and pine nuts in a food processor container. Purée until a fine paste forms. Add the cheese, olive oil and pepper. Process until puréed. May be stored in a tightly covered container in the refrigerator for several weeks. May add ½ bunch stemmed parsley and/or 1 to 2 cups drained frozen spinach if the pesto is too strong.

Yield: 2 to 3 cups

Mayor Vincent A. Cianci, Jr.'s Marinara Sauce

This is a natural fresh sauce that can be used as the base for a meat sauce, a pink sauce or Clam Zuppa.

6 cloves of garlic, crushed
1/4 cup extra-virgin olive oil
2 large red onions, chopped
10 pounds plum tomatoes, blanched
2 large carrots, chopped

1/2 cup finely chopped fresh parsley
1/2 cup chopped fresh basil
1/2 cup dry red wine (optional)
1/2 cup grated Parmesan cheese
Salt and pepper to taste

Sauté the garlic in the olive oil in a saucepan over medium heat just until tender. Add the onions. Sauté until the onions are translucent. Process the tomatoes through a food mill into the onion mixture. Mix in the remaining ingredients. Simmer for 2 to 6 hours or until thickened. Adjust the seasonings. Serve over pasta.

Yield: 16 cups

Sun-Dried Tomato Sauce

2 shallots, chopped
1 teaspoon crushed garlic
1/8 teaspoon crushed pepper seeds
1 teaspoon crushed basil
Salt and black pepper to taste
Virgin olive oil

1 can chicken broth
3 drops of soy sauce, or to taste
1/2 jar sun-dried tomato purée
Julienned sun-dried tomatoes
1 small jar roasted
red peppers, puréed

Sauté the first 6 ingredients in a skillet coated with olive oil over medium-high heat until the shallots are translucent. Add the chicken broth. Cook for 15 minutes or until the sauce is somewhat reduced. Add the soy sauce, tomato purée, tomato strips and red peppers. Cook for 5 minutes longer. Toss with pasta to serve.

Yield: 2 to 3 cups

Éntrées

"Many days we were so wiped out after spending time in the nursery, we would go back to the House and sit in the kitchen. Pretty soon someone would come in, whether it was another person in a similar situation or a volunteer, and we would start talking. The tension would ease and go away."

—Larry Orlando, parent

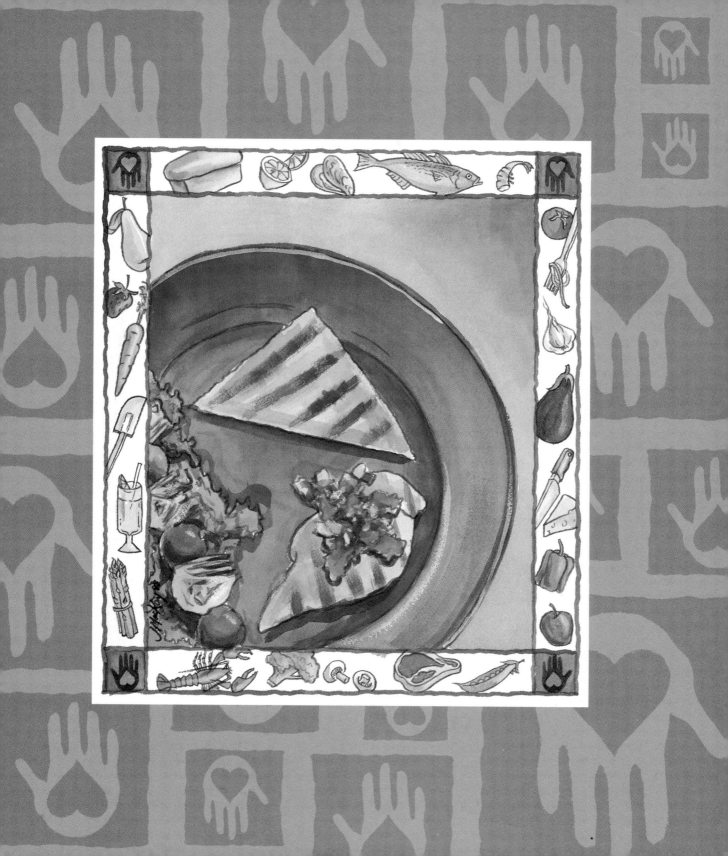

Entrées

Mushroom and Spinach-Stuffed
Beef Tenderloin 101

Sliced Steak with Mustard Sauce 102

Beef Bourguignon 103

Beef Fillets with Mozzarella Cheese 104

French Meat Pie 105

Kids' Kasserole 106

Veal Parmigiana 107

Veal Scaloppine with
Mushrooms 108

Lamb with Garlic and Rosemary 109

Mediterranean Lamb Chops 110

Crown Roast of Pork with
Apricot Bread Stuffing 111

Pork with Pear Chutney 112

Marinated Pork Tenderloins with
Sour Cream Mustard Sauce 113

Cajun-Style Pork Chops 114

Pork Cutlets with Apples, Parsnips
and Cabbage 115

Raspberry Pork Chops 116

Sausage and Mushrooms with
Creamy Polenta 117

Roasted Chicken with Peppers
and Potatoes 118

Chicken Mexicana 119

Company Chicken 120

Chicken Dijon 121

Baked Chicken Breasts with
Gruyère Cheese and Mushrooms 122

Chicken Marsala 123

Bleu Cheese-Stuffed Chicken 124

Stir-Fry Chicken 125

Chicken Cordon Bleu 126

South County Chicken Pie 127

Almond Chicken 128

Eggplant Turkey Casserole 129

Barley and Turkey Stuffed Peppers 130

Mango Chutney 131

Szechuan Peanut Sauce 131

Mushroom and Spinach-Stuffed Beef Tenderloin

1 tablespoon margarine
3 cups sliced shiitake mushroom caps
1/2 cup chopped shallots
2 tablespoons brandy
1 teaspoon olive oil
8 cups torn spinach
1 clove of garlic, minced
1/4 teaspoon salt

1/4 teaspoon pepper
1 (4-pound) beef tenderloin,
fat trimmed
1/4 teaspoon salt
1/4 teaspoon pepper
1 teaspoon olive oil
1/2 teaspoon salt
1/4 teaspoon pepper

Melt the margarine in a large nonstick skillet over medium-high heat. Add the mushroom caps and shallots. Sauté for 4 minutes. Add the brandy. Cook for 30 seconds or until the brandy has evaporated. Spoon into a large bowl and set aside.

Heat 1 teaspoon olive oil in a skillet over medium heat. Add the spinach and garlic. Sauté for 30 seconds or until the spinach is wilted. Remove the spinach to a colander and press with a spoon until barely moist. Add the spinach, 1/4 teaspoon salt and 1/4 teaspoon pepper to the mushroom mixture; mix well and set aside.

To butterfly the tenderloin, slice lengthwise to but not through the other side. Open the halves, laying the tenderloin flat. Slice each half lengthwise to but not through the other side; open flat. Place heavy-duty plastic wrap over the tenderloin and pound to an even thickness with a meat mallet or rolling pin. Remove and discard the plastic wrap.

Sprinkle 1/4 teaspoon salt and 1/4 teaspoon pepper over the tenderloin. Spread the spinach mixture over the center of the tenderloin, leaving a 1/2-inch margin on each side. Fold over 3 or 4 inches of the small end. Roll up from the short end as for a jelly roll. Secure with kitchen string at 2-inch internals. Brush the tenderloin with 1 teaspoon olive oil. Sprinkle with 1/2 teaspoon salt and 1/4 teaspoon pepper.

Spray the rack of a broiler pan with nonstick cooking spray. Place the tenderloin on the rack in the pan. Bake at 500 degrees for 35 minutes or until a meat thermometer inserted in the thickest part of the tenderloin registers 160 degrees for medium. Let stand for 10 minutes before slicing. Serve warm or chilled.

Yield: 4 to 6 servings

Sliced Steak with Mustard Sauce

1 (2-pound) flank steak
2 tablespoons flour
1 large onion, chopped

2 tablespoons butter
Mustard Sauce

Cut the steak into 1/2-inch slices. Coat the slices with the flour. Cook the onion in the butter in a skillet for 5 minutes or until browned. Add the steak. Cook for 5 minutes or until browned. Reduce the heat. Cook, covered, for 20 minutes or until the steak reaches the desired degree of doneness. Add the Mustard Sauce, tossing to coat. Serve immediately.

Yield: 4 to 6 servings

Mustard Sauce

1/4 cup butter
3 tablespoons flour
1 1/2 tablespoons cider vinegar or
red wine vinegar
1 tablespoon dry mustard
1 teaspoon paprika

1/2 teaspoon thyme
1/2 teaspoon salt
1/2 teaspoon black pepper
1/2 teaspoon cayenne
1 cup water

Melt the butter in a saucepan. Stir in the flour. Cook until heated through but not browned, stirring constantly. Add the vinegar, mustard, paprika, thyme, salt, black pepper, cayenne and water and mix well. Simmer for 20 minutes or until the mixture is heated through and the flavors have blended.

Beef Bourguignon

Salt pork or lean bacon, cut into pieces
3 pounds lean stew beef, cut into
2- to 3-inch pieces
3 cups burgundy
2 cups beef bouillon
1 tablespoon tomato paste
2 to 3 cloves of garlic, crushed

1/2 teaspoon thyme
1 bay leaf
Salt to taste
Pepper to taste
Flour
Chopped onion
Sliced mushrooms

Brown a small amount of salt pork in a skillet. Remove the salt pork and set aside. Brown a few beef cubes at a time in the drippings in the skillet. Use a slotted spoon to remove the beef cubes to a casserole or Dutch oven as they finish browning.

Drain the skillet well. Add the burgundy to the skillet, stirring to scrape up the browned bits. Add the burgundy and salt pork to the beef cubes in the casserole. Add the beef bouillon. Stir in the tomato paste, garlic, thyme, bay leaf, salt and pepper. Bake, covered, at 325 degrees for 2 1/2 to 3 hours or until the beef is tender.

Remove from the oven. Remove and discard the bay leaf. Stir enough flour into the stew to thicken to the desired consistency. Stir in chopped onion and sliced mushrooms to taste. Return to the oven. Bake until heated through. Serve over noodles or rice.

Yield: 4 to 6 servings

Beef Fillets with Mozzarella Cheese

4 (1/2-inch-thick) beef fillets
2 tablespoons olive oil
Salt and pepper to taste
2 tomatoes, cut into halves crosswise

2 tablespoons chopped parsley
1 clove of garlic, minced
1 teaspoon basil flakes
4 slices mozzarella cheese

Flatten each fillet with a meat mallet or rolling pin. Heat the olive oil in a skillet. Add the fillets. Cook until the fillets reach the desired degree of doneness. Season with salt and pepper. Remove the fillets and arrange in a single layer in a shallow baking pan.

Fry the tomatoes in the drippings in the skillet until lightly browned. Place 1 tomato half cut side up on each fillet. Season with additional salt and pepper.

Combine the parsley, garlic and basil in a bowl and mix well. Sprinkle generously over the tomatoes. Place 1 slice of cheese over each fillet. Bake at 375 degrees for 10 to 15 minutes or until the cheese is melted. Serve immediately.

Yield: 4 servings

From the Heart...

"Guard well within yourself that treasure, kindness. Know how to give without hesitation, how to lose without regret, how to acquire without meanness."
—George Sand

...of Our House

French Meat Pie

1 pound ground beef
8 ounces ground pork
1/2 cup finely chopped onion
1/2 cup water
2 large potatoes, peeled,
cut into quarters
1/2 teaspoon salt

1/4 teaspoon allspice
1/4 teaspoon ground cloves
1/8 teaspoon pepper
1 recipe (2-crust) pie pastry
1 egg yolk
2 tablespoons water

Combine the ground beef, ground pork, onion and 1/2 cup water in a medium saucepan and mix well. Cook, covered, over low heat until the ground beef and pork are cooked through, stirring occasionally.

Boil the potatoes in water to cover in a small saucepan until tender; drain. Add to the meat mixture. Add the salt, allspice, cloves and pepper and mix well. Remove from the heat. Mash the mixture with a potato masher.

Roll the pastry into two 11-inch circles on a lightly floured surface. Fit 1 pastry into a 9-inch pie plate. Fill with the meat mixture. Cover with the remaining pastry, fluting the edge and cutting several vents.

Brush the top pastry with a mixture of the egg yolk and 2 tablespoons water. Bake at 450 degrees for 20 minutes or until the crust is golden brown.

Yield: 6 servings

Kids' Kasserole

1 pound ground beef
1 medium onion, minced
1 green bell pepper, minced
1 (28-ounce) can chopped tomatoes
1 tablespoon Worcestershire sauce

1 teaspoon dried oregano
Salt to taste
4 cups medium egg noodles
1½ cups shredded Cheddar cheese

Brown the ground beef in a large skillet over medium heat, stirring until crumbly; drain well. Increase the heat to high. Add the onion and green pepper. Cook for 5 minutes, stirring constantly. Add the undrained tomatoes, Worcestershire sauce, oregano and salt to the meat mixture and mix well. Bring to a boil; reduce the heat to low. Simmer while the noodles are cooking.

Bring a large saucepan of water to a boil. Add the noodles. Cook for 6 minutes or until very tender; drain well. Return the noodles to the saucepan. Add the meat mixture and mix well. Spoon the noodle mixture into a casserole. Top with the cheese. Bake at 350 degrees for 10 to 20 minutes or until the mixture is heated through and the cheese is melted.

Yield: 6 servings

From the Heart...

"Where we love is home. Home that our feet may leave but not our hearts."
—Oliver Wendell Holmes, Jr.

...of Our House

$\mathcal{V}$eal Parmigiana

1 pound thin veal scallops
2 eggs, beaten
1 cup seasoned dry bread crumbs
1/2 cup (about) olive oil or vegetable oil

Tomato Sauce
1 (8-ounce) package sliced
mozzarella cheese
1/4 cup grated Parmesan cheese

Wipe the veal with damp paper towels. Dip the veal into the eggs, then coat lightly with the bread crumbs. Heat 1/4 cup of the olive oil in a large skillet. Add the veal a few slices at a time. Cook for 2 to 3 minutes per side or until golden brown, adding additional olive oil if needed. Layer the veal, Tomato Sauce, mozzarella cheese and Parmesan cheese 1/2 at a time in a 6x10-inch baking dish, ending with Parmesan cheese. Bake, covered with foil, at 350 degrees for 30 minutes or until bubbly.

Yield: 4 to 6 servings

Tomato Sauce

2 tablespoons olive oil or vegetable oil
1/2 cup chopped onion
1 clove of garlic, crushed
1 (17-ounce) can Italian tomatoes
2 teaspoons sugar

3/4 teaspoon salt
1/2 teaspoon dried oregano
1/4 teaspoon dried basil
1/4 teaspoon pepper

Heat the olive oil in a medium saucepan. Add the onion and garlic. Sauté for 5 minutes or until golden brown. Add the undrained tomatoes, sugar, salt, oregano, basil and pepper and mix well. Simmer for 5 minutes.

Veal Scaloppine with Mushrooms

1 ounce dried porcini mushrooms
2 cups warm water
1¹/2 pounds (¹/4-inch) veal cutlets,
cut into halves
1 teaspoon salt
¹/4 teaspoon pepper
3 tablespoons flour
2 tablespoons olive oil
1 small onion, chopped
1 clove of garlic, minced

8 ounces any fresh mushrooms,
thinly sliced
1 cup chicken stock or chicken broth
1 tablespoon minced fresh sage, or
1 teaspoon dried
1 tablespoon minced fresh parsley
2 tablespoons butter
1 tablespoon olive oil
¹/2 cup dry red wine
¹/4 to ¹/2 cup chicken stock

Soak the porcini mushrooms in the warm water for 20 to 30 minutes or until softened. Remove the mushrooms; rinse well and chop coarsely. Strain the soaking liquid into a bowl. Add the porcini mushrooms and set aside. Season the veal with the salt and pepper. Dust lightly with the flour and set aside.

Heat 2 tablespoons olive oil in a large skillet over medium heat. Add the onion and garlic. Cook for 2 to 3 minutes or until tender. Stir in the fresh mushrooms. Add 1 cup chicken stock, undrained porcini mushrooms, sage and parsley and mix well. Simmer for 5 minutes.

Heat the butter and 1 tablespoon olive oil in a large nonreactive skillet over medium heat until the butter is melted. Add the veal slices. Cook for 1 to 2 minutes or until lightly browned, turning once. Stir in the wine and ¹/4 to ¹/2 cup chicken stock. Simmer for 3 minutes or until slightly reduced. Add the mushroom mixture and mix well. Simmer for 2 minutes.

Yield: 4 servings

Lamb with Garlic and Rosemary

Have your butcher butterfly a leg of lamb so that it forms one boneless piece. The lamb is best when it is marinated for the full two days.

1 small onion, finely chopped
6 cloves of garlic, minced
2 teaspoons chopped fresh rosemary
Grated peel and juice of 1 lemon

1 cup red wine
1 teaspoon salt
1 (4-pound) leg of lamb

Combine the onion, garlic, rosemary, lemon peel, lemon juice, wine and salt in a nonreactive dish just large enough to hold the lamb; mix well. Add the lamb, turning to coat well. Marinate, covered with plastic wrap, in the refrigerator for 4 hours to 2 days, turning occasionally.

Remove the lamb from the marinade, reserving the remaining marinade. Broil 4 inches from the heat source for 15 to 20 minutes per side or until a meat thermometer inserted in the thickest part of the lamb registers 145 degrees for medium rare, brushing occasionally with the reserved marinade. Garnish with sprigs of fresh rosemary. Serve with Cold Weather Roasted Vegetables (page 147) and warm garlic bread. May be grilled instead of broiled.

Yield: 4 to 6 servings

$\mathcal{M}$editerranean Lamb Chops

Lamb is wonderful when marinated, then roasted in the oven or grilled or broiled. Leftover lamb can be made into sandwiches or used in salads.

2 cloves of garlic, minced
1 teaspoon minced fresh or
dried rosemary
1/2 cup olive oil
1/4 cup red wine vinegar

1/2 teaspoon salt
1/4 teaspoon freshly ground pepper
4 (12-ounce) lamb chops
1/4 cup olive oil

Combine the garlic, rosemary, 1/2 cup olive oil, vinegar, salt and pepper in a large nonreactive shallow dish and whisk until mixed. Add the lamb chops, turning to coat well. Marinate, covered, in the refrigerator for 2 to 24 hours.

Remove the lamb chops from the marinade, discarding the remaining marinade. Heat 1/4 cup olive oil in a large skillet. Add the lamb chops. Cook for 3 minutes per side or until the lamb chops reach the desired degree of doneness.

Yield: 4 servings

Crown Roast of Pork with Apricot Bread Stuffing

For a great harvest dinner, serve stuffed pumpkin appetizers before bringing this eye-catching and tantalizing roast to the table.

1 (17-ounce) can apricots
1/2 cup margarine
1/2 yellow onion, finely chopped
3 ribs celery, finely chopped
2 (10-ounce) cans chicken broth

1 (6-ounce) package stuffing mix
1 (8-rib) crown pork roast
1/4 teaspoon salt
1/4 teaspoon pepper
1/4 teaspoon dillweed

Drain the apricots, reserving the juice. Chop the apricots and set aside. Melt the margarine in a large skillet. Add the onion and celery. Sauté for 5 minutes or until tender. Add the apricots. Sauté briefly. Add the chicken broth and stuffing mix and mix well. Stir in the reserved apricot juice.

Place the roast in a roasting pan sprayed with nonstick cooking spray. Sprinkle with the salt, pepper and dill. Stuff the cavity with the apricot mixture. Cover the cavity with foil.

Bake at 350 degrees for 1 1/2 to 2 hours or until cooked through. Remove the foil during the last 20 minutes baking time.

Yield: 8 servings

Pork with Pear Chutney

1/4 cup packed brown sugar
1 tablespoon cider vinegar
1 teaspoon Dijon mustard
2 (1 1/2-pound) pork tenderloins

1/4 teaspoon salt
1/4 teaspoon pepper
Pear Chutney

Combine the brown sugar, vinegar and Dijon mustard in a bowl and mix well. Rub the tenderloins with the salt and pepper. Place the tenderloins on a rack in a broiler pan.

Broil 7 inches from the heat source for 8 minutes. Turn the tenderloin over and brush with some of the brown sugar mixture. Broil for 8 minutes longer and glaze again. Broil for 2 minutes longer or until the pork is cooked through.

Let the tenderloins stand for several minutes before slicing thinly. Spoon Pear Chutney over the tenderloins to serve.

Yield: 6 servings

Pear Chutney

1 (28-ounce) can pear halves
1/3 cup pickled sweet peppers
1/4 cup raisins or currants
1 teaspoon brown sugar
2 teaspoons cider vinegar

1/4 teaspoon ginger
1/4 teaspoon salt
1/4 teaspoon pepper
1 green onion, chopped

Drain the pears, reserving 1/2 cup juice. Cut the pears into 1/2-inch chunks. Combine the reserved juice, peppers, raisins, brown sugar, vinegar, ginger, salt and pepper in a 2-quart saucepan. Bring to a boil; reduce the heat. Simmer for 5 minutes. Stir in the pears and green onion. Cook for 5 minutes.

$\mathcal{M}$arinated Pork Tenderloins with Sour Cream Mustard Sauce

¹/2 cup soy sauce
¹/2 cup bourbon
¹/4 cup packed brown sugar

3 (12-ounce) pork tenderloins
Sour Cream Mustard Sauce

Combine the soy sauce, bourbon and brown sugar in a shallow dish and mix well. Add the tenderloins, turning to coat well. Marinate, covered, in the refrigerator for several hours to overnight. Remove the tenderloins from the marinade, reserving the remaining marinade. Place the tenderloins in a baking pan. Bake at 325 degrees for 45 minutes or until cooked through, basting frequently with the reserved marinade. Serve with Sour Cream Mustard Sauce.

Yield: 4 servings

Sour Cream Mustard Sauce

¹/2 cup sour cream
¹/2 cup mayonnaise
1 tablespoon dry mustard

1 tablespoon chopped
scallions or onion
1¹/2 tablespoons white wine vinegar

Combine the sour cream, mayonnaise, mustard, scallions and vinegar in a medium bowl and mix well. Let stand at room temperature for 4 hours or longer.

Cajun-Style Pork Chops

2 tablespoons butter
4 thick boneless pork chops, or
1¼ pounds boneless
pork shoulder, sliced
1 teaspoon salt
¼ teaspoon cayenne
⅓ cup finely chopped onion
2 cloves of garlic, minced

1 bay leaf
1 teaspoon paprika
½ teaspoon black pepper
½ teaspoon dried thyme
½ cup chicken broth
½ cup white wine
¾ to 1 cup sour cream

Heat a small amount of the butter in a large skillet. Add the pork chops. Cook until browned on both sides. Sprinkle with the salt and cayenne. Remove the pork chops from the skillet and set aside.

Add the remaining butter to the skillet. Add the onion and garlic. Sauté until tender but not browned. Add the bay leaf, paprika, black pepper and thyme and mix well. Add the chicken broth and wine. Bring to a simmer. Return the pork chops to the skillet. Simmer, covered, over medium heat for 20 minutes. Remove the pork chops to serving plates.

Add the sour cream to the onion mixture in the skillet and mix gently. Cook over low heat until heated through, stirring frequently. Season with additional salt and black pepper. Remove and discard bay leaf. Spoon the sauce over the pork chops. Serve with steamed rice and broccoli.

Yield: 4 servings

$\mathcal{P}$ork Cutlets with Apples, Parsnips and Cabbage

2 tablespoons vegetable oil
2 small pork cutlets
2 medium parsnips, peeled,
cut diagonally into 1/3-inch slices
1 McIntosh apple, peeled, cored,
cut into 10 wedges

1/2 small head cabbage,
cored, shredded
1 teaspoon dried basil
Salt and pepper to taste
1/4 cup apple juice

Heat the oil in an ovenproof skillet over medium-high heat. Add the pork cutlets. Cook until browned on both sides. Reduce the heat to medium. Remove the pork cutlets and set aside.

Add the parsnips to the skillet. Sauté until tender-crisp. Add the apple and cabbage. Sauté until the apple is almost tender. Add the basil, salt and pepper and mix well. Add the apple juice and mix well.

Arrange the pork cutlets over the apple mixture. Spoon the pan drippings from the skillet over the cutlets. Bake at 350 degrees for 15 minutes or until the cutlets are cooked through. May substitute sauerkraut or coarsely chopped escarole for the cabbage. May melt low-fat Alpine lace cheese over the cutlets.

Yield: 2 servings

Raspberry Pork Chops

4 lean pork chops
2 tablespoons flour
1½ tablespoons butter
1 tablespoon vegetable oil

6 tablespoons raspberry vinegar
¾ cup chicken broth
½ cup whipping cream

Coat the pork chops with the flour. Heat the butter and oil in a large skillet until the butter is melted. Add the pork chops. Cook until browned on both sides. Remove the pork chops and set aside.

Add the vinegar and chicken broth to the skillet. Cook over low heat until heated through, stirring frequently to scrape up the browned bits. Return the pork chops to the skillet. Simmer for 10 minutes per side. Remove the pork chops to a platter.

Increase the heat to high. Boil the broth mixture in the skillet for 5 minutes or until slightly thickened. Reduce the heat. Add the whipping cream. Cook until thickened, stirring constantly.

Spoon the cream sauce over the pork chops. Serve immediately. May substitute boneless chicken for the pork chops.

Yield: 2 servings

From the Heart...

"We must not only give what we have; we must also give what we are."
—Desire-Joseph Mercier

...of Our House

Sausage and Mushrooms with Creamy Polenta

1 pound sweet Italian sausage,
casings removed
1 pound mushrooms, sliced
1 medium onion, chopped
2 cloves of garlic, minced
1/4 teaspoon pepper

1 (28-ounce) can Italian tomatoes
2 1/2 cups milk
2 cups cornmeal
1 (14-ounce) can chicken broth
1/2 cup grated Parmesan cheese
2 tablespoons chopped fresh parsley

Brown the sausage in a 12-inch skillet over medium heat, stirring until crumbly; drain well, reserving 1 tablespoon drippings.

Cook the mushrooms, onion, garlic and pepper in the reserved drippings in the skillet for 10 minutes or until the liquid has evaporated and the onion and garlic are golden brown, stirring occasionally. Stir in the undrained tomatoes. Bring to a boil. Add the sausage; reduce the heat to low. Simmer until the polenta has finished cooking.

For the polenta, pour the milk into a large saucepan. Add the cornmeal, whisking until smooth. Cook over medium heat until heated through. Combine the chicken broth with enough water to measure 5 cups in a large saucepan. Bring to a boil. Add the chicken broth to the cornmeal mixture. Cook until thickened, stirring constantly. Stir in the cheese. Serve the polenta in a ring around the sausage mixture or in a separate bowl. Sprinkle with the parsley.

Yield: 4 to 6 servings

Roasted Chicken with Peppers and Potatoes

4 shallots, peeled, blanched,
cut into quarters
1/2 red bell pepper, cut into strips
1/2 green bell pepper, cut into strips
1 pound red potatoes, cut into cubes
1 teaspoon dried rosemary
3 cloves of garlic, minced

3 tablespoons olive oil
Salt to taste
Pepper to taste
1 chicken breast with bone,
cut into halves
1 tablespoon lemon juice
1/2 cup chicken broth

Combine the shallots, red pepper, green pepper, potatoes, rosemary and garlic in a large bowl. Add 2 to 2 1/2 tablespoons of the olive oil and toss well. Season with salt and pepper. Spoon into a large casserole.

Rub the chicken with the lemon juice, remaining olive oil, salt and pepper. Arrange the chicken over the vegetable mixture. Bake at 450 degrees for 20 minutes. Reduce the oven temperature to 375 degrees. Bake for 15 minutes or until the chicken is cooked through.

Remove the chicken and vegetables to a platter. Add the chicken broth to the casserole. Cook for 1 minute, stirring frequently to scrape up the browned bits. Spoon over the chicken.

Yield: 2 servings

Chicken Mexicana

6 boneless skinless chicken breasts
1/4 cup melted margarine or butter
1 teaspoon salt
1/2 teaspoon paprika
1/8 teaspoon pepper, or to taste
6 ounces tortilla chips
1 (10-ounce) can enchilada sauce

1 cup shredded Cheddar cheese
1 (4-ounce) can chopped green
chiles, drained
1/2 cup chopped green onions
1 (4-ounce) can black olives, drained,
pitted, sliced (optional)

Arrange the chicken in a single layer in a 9x13-inch baking pan. Spoon the melted margarine over the chicken. Sprinkle with the salt, paprika and pepper. Bake at 350 degrees for 35 to 45 minutes or until the chicken is cooked through. Remove from the oven.

Crumble the tortilla chips over the chicken. Spoon the enchilada sauce over the top. Sprinkle with the cheese, green chiles, green onions and olives. Bake for 15 minutes or until the cheese is melted. Remove to serving plates with a slotted spoon.

Yield: 6 servings

Company Chicken

This is a very rich but very tasty dish. Serve it with rice and a salad for a complete meal. Any unused bread crumb mixture can be frozen for later use.

2 cups fresh bread crumbs
1/2 cup grated Parmesan cheese
1/2 cup chopped parsley
1 teaspoon garlic powder, or to taste
1 teaspoon pepper, or to taste

8 chicken breasts, split into halves,
skin removed, deboned
1/2 cup melted butter
Lemon Pepper Sauce

Mix the bread crumbs, cheese, parsley, garlic powder and pepper in a bowl. Dip the chicken into the butter, then into the bread crumb mixture. Arrange the chicken in a single layer in a shallow baking dish. Bake at 375 degrees for 20 to 25 minutes or until the chicken is cooked through. Spoon Lemon Pepper Sauce over the chicken during the last 5 minutes baking time.

Yield: 10 to 12 servings

Lemon Pepper Sauce

1/2 cup melted butter
1/4 cup lemon juice
2 whole cloves of garlic

1/2 teaspoon lemon pepper
1 teaspoon salt

Combine the butter, lemon juice, garlic, lemon pepper and salt in a saucepan. Boil for 5 minutes. Remove and discard the garlic.

Chicken Dijon

3 tablespoons butter
4 chicken breasts, split into halves,
skin removed, deboned
1 tablespoon cornstarch
1 cup chicken broth

½ cup light cream
2 tablespoons Dijon mustard
2 tomatoes, cut into wedges (optional)
2 tablespoons minced
fresh parsley (optional)

Melt the butter in a large skillet. Add the chicken. Cook for 20 minutes or until browned. Remove the chicken and keep warm.

Stir the cornstarch into the drippings in the skillet. Cook for 1 minute, stirring constantly. Add the chicken broth and cream. Stir in the Dijon mustard. Return the chicken to the skillet. Cook for 10 minutes. Remove the chicken to a platter. Top with the tomato wedges and parsley. Serve with rice.

Yield: 4 servings

From the Heart...

"The simplest and shortest ethical precept is to be served by others as little as possible, and to serve others as much as possible."
—Leo Tolstoy

...of Our House

Baked Chicken Breasts with Gruyère Cheese and Mushrooms

2 to 3 chicken breasts, skin
removed, deboned
4 eggs, beaten
Salt to taste
1 cup fine bread crumbs

1/2 cup butter
1/2 pound fresh mushrooms
4 ounces Gruyère cheese, shredded
1 cup chicken stock
Juice of 1 lemon

Cut the chicken into strips. Combine the eggs and salt in a large bowl and mix well. Add the chicken. Marinate, covered, in the refrigerator for 1 hour.

Remove the chicken from the marinade, discarding the remaining marinade. Coat the chicken with the bread crumbs. Cook the chicken in the butter in a small skillet until lightly browned. Remove to a 1 1/2-quart casserole.

Slice the mushrooms over the chicken. Sprinkle with the cheese. Pour the chicken stock over the chicken. Bake at 350 degrees for 30 minutes or until the chicken is cooked through. Spoon the lemon juice over the chicken just before serving.

Yield: 2 to 3 servings

Chicken Marsala

2 pounds boneless skinless
chicken breasts
1/4 cup grated Parmesan cheese
1 teaspoon salt
1/4 teaspoon pepper
1/4 to 1/2 teaspoon finely
chopped garlic
1/4 to 1/2 teaspoon paprika

1/4 to 1/2 teaspoon thyme
1 tablespoon parsley
1/3 cup bread crumbs
2 teaspoons vegetable oil
1/4 cup melted margarine
2 teaspoons vegetable oil
1/3 cup marsala

Trim all visible fat from the chicken; cut the chicken into large serving pieces. Combine the cheese, salt, pepper, garlic, paprika, thyme, parsley and bread crumbs in a bowl and toss to mix.

Pour 2 teaspoons oil and a small amount of water into a 9x13-inch baking pan sprayed with nonstick cooking spray. Coat the chicken with some of the bread crumb mixture. Arrange the chicken in a single layer in the baking pan. Top with the remaining crumb mixture. Sprinkle with the melted margarine and 2 teaspoons oil.

Bake at 350 degrees for 35 minutes. Remove from the oven. Pour the wine over and around the chicken. Cover tightly with foil. Reduce the oven temperature to 325 or 300 degrees. Bake for 5 to 10 minutes or until the chicken is cooked through. Spoon pan drippings over the chicken to serve.

Yield: 4 to 8 servings

Bleu Cheese-Stuffed Chicken

4 large boneless skinless
chicken breast halves
Salt and pepper to taste
3 ounces cream cheese, softened
1/4 cup crumbled bleu cheese

1/2 cup toasted chopped pecans
2 tablespoons melted
margarine or butter
1/4 teaspoon paprika

Place each piece of chicken between 2 sheets of plastic wrap. Flatten each 1/4 inch thick with a meat mallet or rolling pin. Remove and discard the plastic wrap. Season the chicken with salt and pepper.

Combine the cream cheese, bleu cheese and pecans in a small bowl and mix well. Place about 1/4 cup of the mixture in the center of 1 chicken piece. Fold the chicken around the filling to form a mound. Repeat with the remaining chicken and cream cheese mixture. Place in a square 2-quart baking dish.

Combine the margarine and paprika in a small bowl. Brush over the chicken. Bake at 350 degrees for 30 minutes or until the chicken is cooked through. Garnish with snipped fresh parsley.

Yield: 4 servings

From the Heart...

"We can do no great things—only small things with great love."
—Mother Teresa

...of Our House

Stir-Fry Chicken

This recipe is easy to adapt to whatever vegetables you happen to have on hand. Simply use more or fewer vegetables to increase or decrease the number of servings. The delicious leftovers can be reheated in a microwave.

1 tablespoon vegetable oil	1 onion, cut into rings
2 teaspoons soy sauce	2 to 3 carrots, thinly sliced
1 teaspoon cornstarch	2 to 3 ribs celery, thinly sliced
1 pound boneless chicken, cut into bite-size pieces	1 green bell pepper, cut into 1-inch pieces
1/2 teaspoon crushed red pepper	1 red bell pepper, cut into 1-inch pieces
1/2 cup chicken broth	8 ounces broccoli, cut into 1-inch pieces
1/2 teaspoon ginger	1 (8-ounce) can sliced water chestnuts, drained
1 tablespoon soy sauce	
2 teaspoons cornstarch	
1/4 cup vegetable oil	
1 clove of garlic, minced	

Mix 1 tablespoon oil, 2 teaspoons soy sauce and 1 teaspoon cornstarch in a small bowl. Add the chicken, stirring to coat. Sprinkle with the red pepper. Marinate, covered, in the refrigerator for 20 minutes. Mix the chicken broth, ginger, 1 tablespoon soy sauce and 2 teaspoons cornstarch in a bowl and set aside.

Remove the chicken from the marinade, discarding the remaining marinade. Heat 1/4 cup oil in a wok or skillet. Add the chicken. Stir-fry until the chicken is cooked through. Remove the chicken and keep warm.

Add the garlic, onion, carrots, celery, green pepper and red pepper to the wok. Stir-fry until the vegetables are tender. Add the broccoli. Stir-fry until the broccoli is tender. Add the water chestnuts, chicken and broth mixture and mix well. Cook until the sauce is thickened, stirring constantly. Serve with rice or crusty bread.

Yield: 4 servings

Chicken Cordon Bleu

2 chicken cutlets
1 egg, beaten
Italian bread crumbs

4 slices mozzarella cheese
4 slices prosciutto
White wine

Dip the cutlets into the egg, then into the bread crumbs. Place 2 slices cheese and 2 slices prosciutto on each cutlet. Roll up each cutlet, securing each with 2 wooden picks.

Place the cutlets in a greased 9x12-inch glass baking dish. Bake, covered, at 400 degrees for 30 minutes. Remove from the oven.

Add enough wine to the baking dish to reach halfway up the chicken rolls. Bake, uncovered, for 30 minutes or until the chicken is cooked through, basting frequently.

Editor's Note: This recipe is easy to increase, but add 1 more egg if serving more than 5. Baking time may need to be adjusted.

Yield: 2 servings

From the Heart...

*"Look up and not down. Look forward and not back.
Look out and not in. Lend a hand."*
—Edward Everett Hale

...of Our House

South County Chicken Pie

1 (4- to 5-pound) chicken	1 teaspoon salt
1 1/2 quarts water	1/2 teaspoon onion salt
1 teaspoon salt	1/2 teaspoon celery salt
1 small onion, chopped	Pepper to taste
1 carrot, chopped	Yellow food coloring (optional)
1 rib celery, chopped	1 recipe (2-crust) pie pastry
1/2 cup flour	

Combine the chicken, water, 1 teaspoon salt, onion, carrot and celery in a large stockpot. Simmer, covered, until the vegetables are tender. Strain the broth into a large bowl. Measure out 3 1/2 cups of the broth, discarding the remainder of the broth or reserving for another use. Remove and discard the chicken skin and bones. Coarsely chop the chicken.

Combine the flour, 1 teaspoon salt, onion salt, celery salt and pepper in a bowl. Add 1/2 cup of the reserved broth gradually, mixing until smooth.

Bring the remaining 3 cups broth to a boil in a saucepan. Add the flour mixture gradually, whisking until smooth. Cook until thickened, stirring constantly until smooth. Stir in food coloring. Add the chicken and mix well.

Fit 1 pastry into a 9-inch deep-dish pie plate. Spoon in the chicken mixture. Top with the remaining pastry, sealing the edge and cutting vents. Bake at 400 degrees for 45 minutes. The chicken mixture may instead be served over rice or open-face biscuits.

Yield: 6 to 8 servings

Almond Chicken

4 cups chopped cooked chicken
³/4 cup light mayonnaise
¹/2 cup cooked rice
1 teaspoon chopped onion
¹/2 cup sliced almonds
1 (10-ounce) can cream of
  mushroom soup

1 cup chopped celery
1 tablespoon lemon juice
1 (4-ounce) can sliced
  mushrooms, drained
1 cup cornflake crumbs
¹/4 cup sliced almonds
2 tablespoons butter

Combine the chicken, mayonnaise, rice, onion, ¹/2 cup almonds, soup, celery, lemon juice and mushrooms in a large bowl and mix well. Spoon into a buttered casserole.

Sprinkle the cornflake crumbs over the chicken mixture. Top with ¹/4 cup almonds. Dot with the butter. Bake at 350 degrees for 30 minutes or until bubbly and heated through. May freeze before baking.

Yield: 8 servings

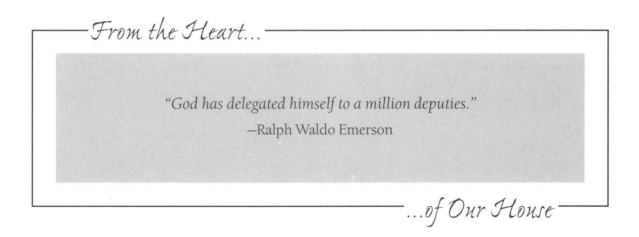

From the Heart...

"God has delegated himself to a million deputies."
–Ralph Waldo Emerson

...of Our House

$\mathcal{E}$ggplant Turkey Casserole

1½ pounds ground turkey
1 onion, chopped
3 cloves of garlic, chopped
1½ eggplant, cut into cubes

1 red bell pepper, chopped
1 green bell pepper, chopped
1 (28-ounce) can crushed tomatoes
Grated Parmesan cheese

Combine the turkey, onion and garlic in a skillet sprayed with nonstick cooking spray. Cook until the onion and garlic are browned, stirring frequently. Combine the eggplant, red pepper, green pepper and undrained tomatoes in a saucepan. Bring to a boil.

Spread the turkey mixture in a 9x13-inch baking pan sprayed with nonstick cooking spray. Sprinkle with Parmesan cheese. Spoon the vegetable mixture over the top.

Bake, covered with foil, for 45 to 50 minutes or until the turkey is cooked through and the vegetables are tender. Remove from the oven. Sprinkle with additional cheese. Bake, uncovered, until the cheese is melted.

Yield: 8 servings

Barley and Turkey Stuffed Peppers

1 cup barley
1 (14-ounce) can low-sodium
chicken broth
1/4 cup water
6 medium green bell peppers
1/3 cup chopped onion
2 tablespoons vegetable oil
1/2 teaspoon chopped garlic
1/2 cup chopped celery

1/2 teaspoon cumin
1 teaspoon dried basil
1 pound ground turkey
1 (8-ounce) can no-salt-added
tomato sauce
Salt and pepper to taste
1 (14-ounce) can crushed or stewed
tomatoes, drained

Combine the barley, chicken broth and water in a saucepan. Bring to a boil; reduce the heat to low. Cook, covered, for 45 minutes or until all the liquid has been absorbed.

Cut the tops off the green peppers and remove the seeds, being careful not to break the peppers. Remove and discard the stems from the tops. Finely chop the tops. Set aside.

Sauté the onion in the oil in a skillet until translucent. Add the garlic, celery and chopped pepper tops. Sauté until the pepper pieces and celery are tender. Add the cumin and basil. Cook for several minutes. Add the turkey. Cook until the turkey is cooked through, stirring frequently. Add the tomato sauce and cooked barley and mix well. Season with salt and pepper.

Fill each pepper with turkey mixture, rounding the tops. Top each with crushed tomatoes. Place in a baking pan or on a baking sheet with sides. Bake at 350 degrees for 30 minutes or until the green peppers are tender.

Editor's Note: These peppers may be prepared 1 day ahead and stored in the refrigerator until needed, but do not top with the tomatoes until ready to reheat and serve.

Yield: 6 servings

Mango Chutney

4 medium mangoes
1/4 cup vinegar
1 tablespoon ginger
1/8 teaspoon cinnamon, or to taste
1 teaspoon salt
1/2 cup Demerara sugar or granulated
light brown sugar

1/2 cup white wine
1/2 teaspoon allspice
1/2 teaspoon cayenne
1 whole clove

Peel and clean the mangoes. Cut the pulp carefully away from the seed. Combine the mango pulp, vinegar, ginger, cinnamon, salt, sugar, wine, allspice, cayenne and clove in a food processor container fitted with a steel blade. Process until puréed. Cook the puréed mixture in a saucepan over low heat for 1 hour or until thickened and greatly reduced. Remove from the heat and let cool. Strain through a fine sieve. Chill for 24 hours before serving. Serve with chicken or fish.

Yield: 8 servings

Szechuan Peanut Sauce

10 tablespoons chunky peanut butter
2 tablespoons low-sodium soy sauce
1 1/2 tablespoons water
2 tablespoons sugar

6 cloves of garlic, minced
4 teaspoons hot chili oil
1 tablespoon finely chopped cilantro

Combine the peanut butter, soy sauce, water, sugar, garlic and oil in a food processor container. Process just until mixed. Stir in the cilantro. Serve with chicken or fish.

Yield: 14 to 16 servings

Vegetables & Side Dishes

"There is a special, special need for a place like a Ronald McDonald House.

Parents will tell you that after three or four days in a hospital, they're utterly

exhausted. The demands of a hospital on parents are so great that you have to make

certain that they can get rest and replenish themselves."

—B. J. Seabury, child life specialist, Director Emeritus,
Child Life, Rhode Island Hospital

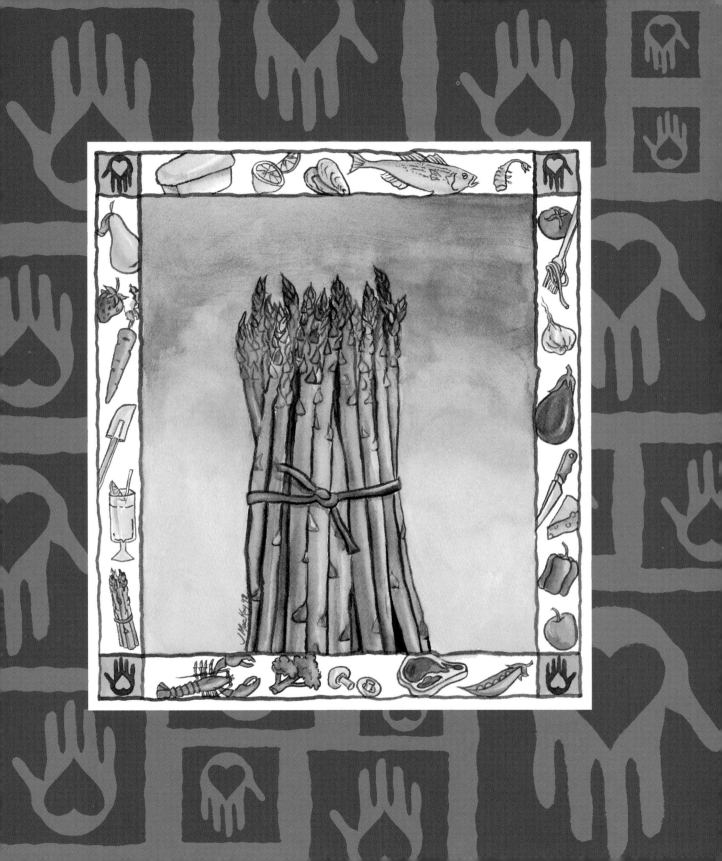

Vegetables & Side Dishes

Asparagus Bundles with Prosciutto 135

Asparagus with Lemon Vinaigrette 136

Bristol's Best Baked Beans 137

Beets with Orange Sauce 138

Copper Carrots 138

Carrot Casserole 139

Corn and Mushroom Bake 139

Baked Eggplant and Feta Cheese 140

Grilled New Potatoes 141

Dijonnaise Potatoes 141

Sautéed Spinach with

Shiitake Mushrooms 142

Quick-and-Easy Sicilian Spinach 143

Squash Soufflé 143

Sweet Potato Streusel Casserole 144

Scalloped Sweet Potatoes

and Apples 145

Lemon Vegetables 145

Julienned Vegetables 146

Cold Weather Roasted Vegetables 147

Buttered Baked Rice 148

Italian Rice and Spinach 148

Risotto with Smoked Mozzarella

and Escarole 149

Asparagus Bundles with Prosciutto

1 pound medium asparagus
4 thin slices prosciutto or ham

3 tablespoons melted butter
1/4 cup grated Parmesan cheese

Cut 2 inches from the stem ends of the asparagus. Scrape the bottom half of each asparagus stalk with a swivel-bladed vegetable peeler. Cook the asparagus in a large saucepan of boiling salted water for 3 to 4 minutes or until tender-crisp. Drain in a colander and rinse under cold running water; drain again.

Divide the asparagus into 4 bundles. Wrap each bundle with a slice of prosciutto, securing with a wooden pick if needed. Arrange the asparagus bundles in an 11x17-inch baking dish.

Drizzle the bundles with the butter. Sprinkle with the cheese. Bake at 375 degrees for 6 to 8 minutes or until the cheese begins to turn golden brown.

Yield: 4 servings

From the Heart...

*"There are in the end three things that last: faith, hope and love,
and the greatest of these is love."*
—St. Paul

...of Our House

Asparagus with Lemon Vinaigrette

1¼ pounds asparagus, trimmed
Lemon Vinaigrette

1 tablespoon finely chopped scallions

Blanch the asparagus in boiling salted water in a large saucepan for 4 minutes or just until tender; drain well. Remove the asparagus to a serving plate. Spoon Lemon Vinaigrette over the asparagus. Sprinkle with the scallions. Serve warm or at room temperature.

Yield: 4 servings

Lemon Vinaigrette

¼ teaspoon finely grated lemon zest
1 tablespoon fresh lemon juice

3 tablespoons extra-virgin olive oil
Salt and freshly ground pepper to taste

Whisk the lemon zest and lemon juice in a small bowl. Whisk in the olive oil gradually. Season with salt and pepper.

Bristol's Best Baked Beans

1 pound small white beans
1/2 teaspoon baking soda
1 cup packed brown sugar
2 tablespoons molasses
1 teaspoon salt

1/4 teaspoon pepper
1/2 teaspoon dry mustard
3 medium onions, chopped
1 (2x2-inch) piece of salt pork,
1/2 inch thick

Soak the beans in water to cover overnight; drain well. Combine the beans with fresh water to cover in a large saucepan Add the baking soda. Boil for 15 minutes, skimming any foam that forms. Drain the beans and rinse well.

Combine the brown sugar, molasses, salt, pepper and dry mustard in a bowl and mix well. Stir in enough boiling water to dissolve the brown sugar.

Combine the beans and brown sugar mixture in a pressure cooker. Add onions and salt pork and mix well. Add enough boiling water to cover; seal. Begin pressure cooking at a medium to high temperature. Reduce the temperature when the pressure cooker begins to hiss. Pressure cook for 35 minutes.

These beans may instead be prepared in a slow cooker or oven. If preparing in a slow cooker, cook on Low for 8 hours or until the beans are tender. If preparing in the oven, bake at 325 degrees for 8 hours or until the beans are tender.

Yield: 6 to 8 servings

$\mathcal{B}$eets with Orange Sauce

¹/4 cup butter
2 tablespoons flour
2 tablespoons light brown sugar
1 cup orange juice

1 teaspoon lemon juice
¹/2 teaspoon salt
1 (16-ounce) can julienned beets

Melt the butter in a saucepan. Stir in the flour. Add the brown sugar, orange juice, lemon juice and salt and mix well. Cook until thickened, stirring occasionally. Stir in the beets.

Yield: 4 servings

$\mathcal{C}$opper Carrots

1 pound carrots, peeled, sliced
1 purple onion, chopped
1 green bell pepper, chopped
1 (10-ounce) can tomato soup
¹/2 cup vegetable oil (optional)
³/4 cup vinegar

1 cup sugar
1 teaspoon prepared mustard
1 teaspoon Worcestershire sauce
1 teaspoon salt
1 teaspoon pepper

Cook the carrots in water to cover in a saucepan until tender-crisp; drain well. Mix the onion, green pepper, soup, oil, vinegar, sugar, mustard, Worcestershire sauce, salt and pepper in a large bowl. Add the carrots and mix well. Marinate, covered, in the refrigerator for 2 to 3 days. Drain well before serving. Serve cold or at room temperature. May substitute canned carrots for the fresh carrots.

Yield: 6 to 8 servings

Carrot Casserole

2 cups thinly sliced carrots
1 cup water
2 Granny Smith apples, thinly sliced
1/2 cup raisins

1/4 cup packed brown sugar or honey
1 1/2 teaspoons cornstarch
1/2 cup orange juice

Cook the carrots in the water in a saucepan for 5 minutes. Add the apples. Cook for 5 minutes; drain well. Combine the carrot mixture, raisins and brown sugar in a bowl. Dissolve the cornstarch in the orange juice and add to the carrot mixture; mix well. Spoon into a buttered 1 1/2-quart casserole. Dot with butter. Bake at 350 degrees for 30 minutes.

Yield: 4 to 6 servings

Corn and Mushroom Bake

1/4 cup flour
1 (16-ounce) can cream-style corn
3 ounces cream cheese, cut into cubes
1/2 teaspoon onion salt
1 (16-ounce) can whole kernel corn, drained

1 (6-ounce) can sliced mushrooms, drained
2 ounces Swiss cheese, shredded
1 1/2 cups soft bread crumbs
3 tablespoons melted butter
1/2 teaspoon Nature's Seasoning

Stir the flour into the cream-style corn in a saucepan. Add the cream cheese and onion salt. Cook until the cream cheese is melted, stirring constantly. Stir the whole kernel corn, mushrooms and Swiss cheese into the hot mixture. Spoon into a 1 1/2-quart casserole. Bake, covered, at 400 degrees for 30 minutes or until heated through. Top with a mixture of the bread crumbs, melted butter and Nature's Seasoning. Bake, uncovered, for 20 minutes or until the bread crumbs are lightly browned. Casserole and bread crumbs may be prepared separately and stored in the refrigerator for up to 1 day before baking.

Yield: 6 to 8 servings

Baked Eggplant and Feta Cheese

1/4 cup olive oil
3 medium eggplant, cut into
1/2-inch slices
1 medium onion, chopped
3 cloves of garlic, chopped
4 red bell peppers, roasted

4 ounces feta cheese
1/2 teaspoon cracked pepper
1 tablespoon chopped fresh oregano
1 teaspoon chopped fresh marjoram
1 cup fresh bread crumbs

Heat 1 tablespoon of the olive oil in a large sauté pan. Add a single layer of eggplant slices. Cook for 2 to 3 minutes per side or until browned. Remove and drain on a baking sheet. Repeat with the remaining eggplant, adding the remaining olive oil as needed.

Place the onion and garlic in the drippings in the sauté pan. Sauté until the mixture becomes fragrant.

Arrange the eggplant in a lightly oiled 9x11-inch baking dish. Top with the onion mixture and red peppers. Crumble the cheese over the top. Sprinkle with the pepper, oregano, marjoram and bread crumbs.

Bake at 350 degrees for 20 to 25 minutes or until golden brown. Serve warm. May be prepared and baked 1 day ahead. May substitute 4 ounces ricotta cheese or 2 ounces ricotta cheese and 2 ounces feta cheese for the 4 ounces feta cheese. May be served as a vegetarian entrée.

Yield: 6 servings

Grilled New Potatoes

4 cups tiny new potatoes
6 tablespoons extra-virgin olive oil
2 tablespoons fresh lemon juice
2 tablespoons minced fresh basil

1 tablespoon minced fresh oregano
1 tablespoon minced fresh rosemary
Salt to taste
Pepper to taste

Boil the potatoes in water to cover in a saucepan for 4 to 6 minutes or just until tender; drain well. Mix the olive oil, lemon juice, basil, oregano, rosemary, salt and pepper in a bowl. Thread the potatoes onto skewers. Brush with the herb mixture. Place the skewers on an oiled grill rack. Grill over medium-high heat for 8 to 12 minutes or until lightly browned and crisp, turning frequently.

Yield: 4 to 6 servings

Dijonnaise Potatoes

4 medium red potatoes,
cut into 3/4-inch cubes
1/4 cup melted butter or margarine
1/2 teaspoon salt

1/2 teaspoon pepper
1 clove of garlic, crushed
1/4 cup Dijon mustard

Arrange the potatoes in a baking dish. Mix the butter, salt, pepper, garlic and Dijon mustard in a bowl. Spoon over the potatoes. Bake at 400 degrees until the potatoes reach the desired degree of doneness. May substitute olive oil or vegetable oil for the melted butter. May add onions, bell peppers or mushrooms.

Yield: 4 servings

Sautéed Spinach with Shiitake Mushrooms

1/2 teaspoon sesame seeds
4 ounces shiitake mushrooms
1 1/2 teaspoons unsalted butter
1 tablespoon olive oil

1/4 teaspoon salt
2 large bunches spinach
Salt to taste
Freshly ground pepper to taste

Cook the sesame seeds in a skillet over medium heat for 5 minutes or until toasted, stirring frequently. Remove and discard the mushroom stems. Thinly slice the mushroom caps.

Heat the butter and olive oil in a large skillet until the butter is melted. Add the mushroom slices. Sprinkle with 1/4 teaspoon salt. Cook for 5 minutes or until tender. Remove to a plate.

Wipe the skillet dry with a paper towel. Trim the stems of the spinach. Rinse the spinach but do not dry. Place the undrained spinach in the skillet. Season with additional salt and pepper. Cook for 7 minutes or until all the liquid has evaporated. Stir in the mushrooms. Cook until the mushrooms are heated through. Remove the spinach mixture to a serving dish. Sprinkle with the toasted sesame seeds.

Yield: 4 servings

From the Heart...

> "If someone listens, or stretches out a hand, or whispers a kind word of encouragement, or attempts to understand a lonely person, extraordinary things begin to happen."
>
> —Loretta Gizarlis

...of Our House

Quick-and-Easy Sicilian Spinach

2 (12-ounce) packages fresh spinach
or 24 ounces baby spinach leaves
4 to 6 cloves of garlic, minced

5 tablespoons olive oil
1 (5-ounce) jar salad olives, drained
Salt and pepper to taste

Wash the spinach and set aside. Sauté the garlic in the olive oil in a large saucepan over medium heat for 3 to 4 minutes or until browned. Add the spinach. Cook over low heat for 6 minutes. Add the olives. Cook for 5 to 8 minutes or until the spinach is tender. Season with salt and pepper.

Yield: 4 to 6 servings

Squash Soufflé

This wonderful vegetable dish is so delicious you might mistake it for dessert. It's especially good for Thanksgiving dinner.

1 (10-ounce) package frozen
squash, thawed
1/2 cup sugar
1/2 cup flour

3 eggs, beaten
2 cups milk
1/4 cup melted butter
Salt, nutmeg and cinnamon to taste

Mix the squash and sugar in a bowl. Add the flour, eggs, milk, butter, salt, nutmeg and cinnamon and mix well. Spoon into a greased 8-inch round or square casserole. Bake at 350 degrees for 50 to 60 minutes or until the squash is tender.

Yield: 4 to 6 servings

Sweet Potato Streusel Casserole

4 large sweet potatoes, baked
1/4 cup melted butter
2 eggs
3/4 cup milk
1/4 cup packed brown sugar
1/3 to 1/2 cup bourbon
1 teaspoon cinnamon

1/2 teaspoon salt
1/8 to 1/4 teaspoon nutmeg
1/2 cup packed brown sugar
1/2 cup rolled oats
1/4 cup flour
1/4 cup butter
3/4 cup finely chopped pecans

Split the sweet potatoes open and scoop the pulp into a large bowl; discard the skins. Beat 1/4 cup melted butter into the sweet potatoes. Beat in the eggs, milk, 1/4 cup brown sugar, bourbon, cinnamon, salt and nutmeg. Spread evenly in a 1 1/2-quart casserole or 8-inch glass baking dish.

Mix 1/2 cup brown sugar, oats and flour in a small bowl. Cut in 1/4 cup butter until crumbly. Stir in the pecans. Sprinkle over the sweet potato mixture.

Bake at 350 degrees for 30 minutes or until heated through. Broil 4 to 5 inches from the heat source for 3 minutes or until browned and bubbly if a crisper topping is desired.

Yield: 6 to 8 servings

From the Heart...

"The best and most beautiful things in the world cannot be seen or even touched. They must be felt with the heart."
—Helen Keller

...of Our House

Scalloped Sweet Potatoes and Apples

6 medium sweet potatoes
1 1/2 cups sliced apples
1/2 cup packed brown sugar

1/2 teaspoon salt
1 teaspoon mace
4 teaspoons butter

Boil the sweet potatoes in water to cover until tender; drain well. Cut into 1/4-inch slices. Place 1 layer of sweet potatoes, then 1 layer of apples in a buttered baking dish. Sprinkle with some of the sugar, salt and mace. Dot with some of the butter. Repeat layers until all ingredients are used, ending with apples. Bake at 350 degrees for 50 minutes.

Yield: 6 to 8 servings

Lemon Vegetables

4 small new potatoes, sliced
2 carrots, cut into thin strips
2 yellow squash, cut into thin strips
1 zucchini, sliced
1/3 cup melted butter or margarine

1 tablespoon grated lemon peel
3 tablespoons lemon juice
1/4 teaspoon salt
1/8 teaspoon pepper

Place the potatoes and carrots in a steamer basket over boiling water. Steam, covered, for 8 minutes. Add the yellow squash and zucchini. Steam, covered, for 2 minutes or until tender-crisp. Remove the vegetable mixture to a large bowl. Mix the butter, lemon peel, lemon juice, salt and pepper in a small bowl. Spoon over the vegetables and toss gently.

Yield: 6 servings

Julienned Vegetables

1 medium yellow squash,
cut into halves
1 medium zucchini, cut into halves
1 medium red bell pepper, julienned
1 medium yellow bell
pepper, julienned

1 medium green bell pepper, julienned
1 medium daikon radish, julienned
1 medium carrot, julienned
$1/2$ cup Basic Vegetable Stock

Scoop the pulp from the yellow squash and zucchini to within $1/4$ inch from the skin. Discard the pulp or reserve for another use. Cut the squash and zucchini peels into julienne strips. Heat a large skillet over medium-high heat. Add all the vegetables and Vegetable Stock. Cook, covered, for 1 to 2 minutes or until tender-crisp.

Yield: 4 servings

Basic Vegetable Stock

6 medium ribs celery, cut into
1-inch pieces
4 medium carrots, cut into
1-inch pieces
4 medium tomatoes, cut into quarters
2 onions, coarsely chopped
1 leek, coarsely chopped

6 sprigs of parsley
2 bay leaves
10 whole black or white peppercorns
$1/2$ cup water
1 (750-ml) bottle dry white wine
$31/2$ cups water

Coarsely chop the celery, carrots and tomatoes separately in a food processor, removing each to a large nonreactive heatproof casserole. Add the onions, leek, parsley, bay leaves, peppercorns and $1/2$ cup water. Cook, tightly covered, over medium-low heat for 30 to 40 minutes or until the vegetables are tender but not browned. Stir in the wine. Increase the heat to medium. Simmer for 45 minutes or until reduced by $1/2$. Add $31/2$ cups water. Simmer for 45 minutes or until reduced by $1/2$ again. Strain through a sieve. Can be frozen in recipe-size portions for up to 3 months. Makes about 6 cups.

$\mathscr{C}$old Weather Roasted Vegetables

Roasted vegetables are quite different from their steamed or boiled counterparts. Roasted, they become sweet and flavorful.

$^1/_3$ cup vegetable oil
12 small red potatoes, cut into halves
3 medium onions, cut into
halves lengthwise
6 carrots, peeled, cut into
halves lengthwise

2 teaspoons chopped rosemary
Salt to taste
Pepper to taste
1 bunch asparagus, trimmed

Spread half the oil in a large baking dish. Arrange the potatoes, onions and carrots in the baking dish. Drizzle with the remaining oil. Sprinkle with the rosemary. Season with salt and pepper.

Bake, covered with foil, at 350 degrees for 30 minutes. Remove from the oven. Turn the vegetables in the baking dish and add the asparagus. Bake, uncovered, for 20 minutes. Serve hot. May add other winter vegetables, such as turnips, parsnips, celery, beets and fennel.

Yield: 4 to 6 servings

Buttered Baked Rice

2 teaspoons salt
2 cups water
1 cup long grain rice
1/3 cup melted butter or margarine

Garlic salt or crushed fresh garlic
to taste
1 (14-ounce) can chicken broth
Chopped parsley
1/4 cup toasted slivered almonds

Bring salted water to a boil in a saucepan. Pour over the rice in a bowl. Let stand for 30 minutes; rinse with cold water and drain well. Combine the rice and butter in a saucepan. Simmer over medium heat for 5 minutes or until the butter is almost absorbed. Spoon into a 1-quart casserole. Sprinkle with garlic salt. Add the chicken broth. Bake, covered, at 325 degrees for 45 minutes. Remove from the oven. Stir in the parsley. Add the almonds. Bake, uncovered, for 10 minutes.

Yield: 4 servings

Italian Rice and Spinach

1 (10-ounce) package frozen spinach
2 cups cooked rice
1/4 cup melted margarine
4 eggs, beaten
1 cup grated Parmesan cheese

1 cup milk
1 tablespoon chopped onion
1 teaspoon salt
1/2 teaspoon thyme
1/2 teaspoon rosemary

Cook the spinach using the package directions; drain well. Mix the spinach, rice, margarine, eggs, cheese, milk, onion, salt, thyme and rosemary in a bowl. Spoon into a 2-quart baking dish. Bake at 350 degrees for 30 minutes. Cut into squares to serve.

Yield: 8 servings

Risotto with Smoked Mozzarella and Escarole

2 tablespoons butter
1/3 cup finely chopped onion
2 cups finely shredded escarole
1 (16-ounce) package arborio rice
1/2 cup dry white wine
4 cups simmering fresh or canned chicken broth

Salt to taste
Freshly ground pepper to taste
1 1/2 cups smoked mozzarella cheese, cut into small cubes
1/4 cup olive oil
1/4 cup freshly grated Parmesan cheese

Melt the butter in a saucepan. Add the onion. Cook until the onion is wilted, stirring constantly. Add the escarole. Cook until the escarole is wilted, stirring constantly.

Add the rice to the escarole mixture. Cook for 1 minute, stirring constantly. Add the wine. Cook for 2 minutes or until all the wine is absorbed, stirring constantly.

Add the simmering chicken broth, salt and pepper to the rice mixture. Cook over medium-high heat for 8 minutes, stirring from the bottom frequently. Add the mozzarella cheese and olive oil. Cook for 1 minute.

Stir in the Parmesan cheese. Cook for 3 to 5 minutes or until thickened and creamy, stirring frequently from the bottom.

Yield: 4 to 6 servings

Desserts

"Thank God for the Ronald McDonald House—its wonderful staff, caring volunteers, and generous supporters. The House provided a safe haven, an environment for us and other families facing similar situations to talk and provide support to one another—something that proved to be far more important than I could ever have imagined."

—Alex Mitchell, parent

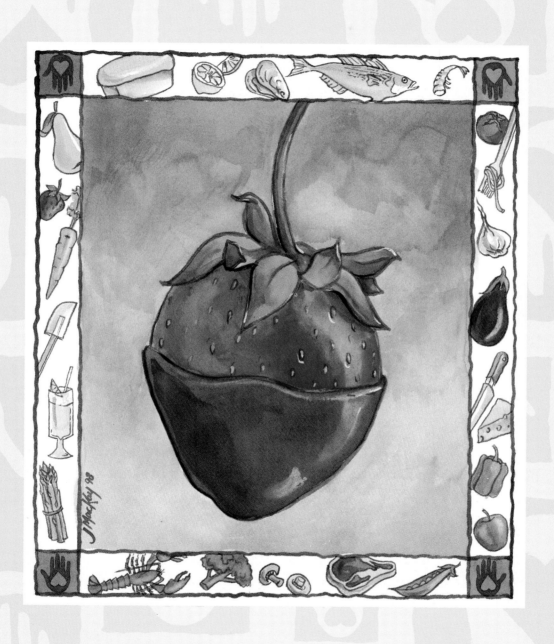

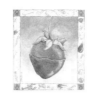

Desserts

Carrot Cake with Cream Cheese
Frosting 153
Chocolate Fudge Cake with
Fudge Frosting 154
White Chocolate Cake 155
Pumpkin Chocolate Chip Cake 156
Hummingbird Cake 156
Apricot Slices 157
Hermits 158
Oatmeal Cookies 158
Orange Cookies 159
Sugar Cookies 160
Martian Cookies 160
Grand Marnier Almond Brownies 161

Sinfully Rich Brownies 162
Cherry Chewbilees 163
Apple Pie 164
French Silk Chocolate Pie 165
Lemonade Pie 165
Chocolate Linzer Tart 166
White Chocolate Cheesecake with
Cranberry Swirl 167
Apple and Oat Pudding 168
Old-Fashioned Baked Custard 168
Tiramisù 169
Blueberry Crisp 170
Strawberries Nirope 170
Baklava 171

Carrot Cake with Cream Cheese Frosting

3 cups flour
2 cups sugar
¹/₂ cup chopped walnuts
2 teaspoons ground cinnamon
2 teaspoons baking powder
1 teaspoon baking soda

2 (16-ounce) cans carrots,
drained, mashed
4 eggs
1¹/₂ cups vegetable oil
Cream Cheese Frosting

Mix the flour, sugar, walnuts, cinnamon, baking powder and baking soda in a large bowl. Mix the carrots and eggs in a medium bowl. Add the oil to the carrot mixture, stirring until mixed. Add the carrot mixture to the dry ingredients and mix well. Spoon the batter into a greased tube pan. Bake at 350 degrees for 1 hour. Cool in the pan for several minutes. Invert onto a plate to cool completely. Spread with Cream Cheese Frosting.

Yield: 16 servings

Cream Cheese Frosting

8 ounces cream cheese, softened
¹/₂ cup margarine, softened
1 teaspoon vanilla extract

1 (1-pound) package
confectioners' sugar

Beat the cream cheese in a mixer bowl until light and fluffy. Beat in the margarine and vanilla. Add the confectioners' sugar gradually, beating until blended and smooth.

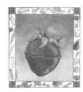

Chocolate Fudge Cake with Fudge Frosting

3 ounces unsweetened chocolate
2¼ cups sifted cake flour
2 teaspoons baking soda
½ teaspoon salt
½ cup butter or margarine, softened
2¼ cups packed light brown sugar

3 eggs
1½ teaspoons vanilla extract
1 cup sour cream
1 cup boiling water
Fudge Frosting

Melt the chocolate in a small heatproof bowl over hot water. Let cool. Sift the flour, baking soda and salt into a large bowl and set aside. Beat the butter in a mixer bowl. Add the brown sugar and eggs and beat for 5 minutes or until light and fluffy. Beat in the vanilla and cooled chocolate. Add the chocolate mixture and sour cream alternately to the flour mixture, beating with a wooden spoon after each addition. Stir in the boiling water; the batter will be thin. Spoon into 3 greased and floured 8-inch cake pans. Bake at 350 degrees for 35 minutes or until the cake springs back when lightly touched. Cool in the pans on a wire rack for 10 minutes. Loosen the edges with a spatula. Remove to a wire rack to cool completely. Spread Fudge Frosting between the layers and over the top and side of the cake.

Yield: 8 to 12 servings

Fudge Frosting

5 ounces unsweetened chocolate
½ cup plus 2 tablespoons butter
1¼ cups confectioners' sugar

½ cup plus 2 tablespoons milk
2½ teaspoons vanilla extract

Melt the chocolate and butter in a small heavy saucepan over low heat. Remove from the heat. Blend the confectioners' sugar, milk and vanilla in a medium bowl. Add the chocolate mixture. Set the bowl in a pan of ice water. Beat with a wooden spoon until of spreading consistency.

White Chocolate Cake

2¹/₂ cups flour
¹/₄ teaspoon baking powder
¹/₄ teaspoon baking soda
¹/₄ teaspoon salt
1 cup butter, softened
2 cups sugar
4 ounces white chocolate, melted

4 eggs
1 cup buttermilk
1 teaspoon vanilla extract
1 cup chopped pecans
1 cup flaked coconut
White Chocolate Frosting

Mix the flour, baking powder, baking soda and salt together and set aside. Cream the butter and sugar in a mixer bowl until light and fluffy. Blend in the white chocolate. Beat in the eggs 1 at a time. Add the flour mixture and buttermilk alternately, beating well after each addition. Fold in the vanilla, pecans and coconut. Spoon into 2 greased and floured 9-inch cake pans. Bake at 350 degrees for 35 to 40 minutes or until the layers test done. Cool in the pans for several minutes. Remove to a wire rack to cool completely. Spread White Chocolate Frosting between the layers and over the top and side of the cake.

Yield: 12 servings

White Chocolate Frosting

3 tablespoons flour
³/₄ cup melted white chocolate
1 cup milk

1 cup butter, softened
1 cup sugar
1¹/₂ teaspoons vanilla extract

Stir the flour into the white chocolate in a saucepan. Blend in the milk gradually. Cook over medium heat until very thick, stirring constantly. Remove from the heat and let cool. Cream the butter and sugar in a large mixer bowl until light and fluffy. Add the vanilla. Add the white chocolate mixture gradually, beating well after each addition until the frosting is the consistency of whipped cream.

Pumpkin Chocolate Chip Cake

4 eggs
1 cup vegetable oil
1 (16-ounce) can pumpkin
2 cups sugar
3 cups flour

2 teaspoons baking powder
2 tablespoons baking soda
1 teaspoon salt
1 teaspoon cinnamon
1 to 2 cups miniature chocolate chips

Mix the eggs, oil, pumpkin, sugar, flour, baking powder, baking soda, salt and cinnamon in a large bowl. Fold in the chocolate chips. Spoon into a 9x13-inch cake pan. Bake at 350 degrees for 50 to 60 minutes or until the cake tests done. The top of the cake may begin to split.

Yield: 15 servings

Hummingbird Cake

3 cups flour
2 cups sugar
1 teaspoon salt
1 teaspoon baking soda
1 teaspoon cinnamon
3 eggs, beaten

1½ cups vegetable oil
1½ teaspoons vanilla extract
1 (8-ounce) can crushed pineapple
2 cups chopped bananas
2 cups chopped pecans or walnuts
Cream Cheese Frosting (page 153)

Combine the flour, sugar, salt, baking soda and cinnamon in a large bowl. Add the eggs and oil and mix well. Add the vanilla, undrained pineapple, bananas and pecans and mix well. Spoon into 3 greased and floured 9-inch cake pans. Bake at 350 degrees for 30 to 40 minutes or until the layers test done. Cool in the pans for several minutes. Remove to a wire rack to cool completely. Spread Cream Cheese Frosting between the layers and over the top and side of the cake.

Yield: 12 to 16 servings

Apricot Slices

2½ cups flour
1 teaspoon baking powder
½ teaspoon baking soda
⅛ teaspoon salt
½ cup melted margarine
1 egg, beaten
½ cup plus 1 tablespoon sour cream

1 jar apricot jam
Sugar to taste
Cinnamon to taste
Flaked coconut
Chopped pecans or walnuts
2 tablespoons sour cream
1 cup confectioners' sugar

Sift the flour, baking powder, baking soda and salt into a large bowl. Add the margarine, egg, and ½ cup plus 1 tablespoon sour cream and mix well. Chill, covered, for 1 hour or longer. Cut the chilled dough into 3 equal portions. Roll each portion into a rectangle on a lightly floured surface. Spread apricot jam over 1 dough portion. Sprinkle with sugar, cinnamon, coconut and pecans. Roll as for a jelly roll. Repeat with the remaining dough.

Place the rolls on a greased cookie sheet. Bake at 350 degrees for 30 minutes or until golden brown. Blend 2 tablespoons sour cream and confectioners' sugar in a bowl. Spread over the warm rolls. Cut into ½- to 1-inch slices.

Yield: 3 dozen

From the Heart...

"Ah! There is nothing like staying at home for real comfort."
—Jane Austen

...of Our House

Hermits

2 cups flour
1 teaspoon cinnamon
1 teaspoon baking soda
1/2 teaspoon salt
3 eggs, beaten

1 1/2 cups packed brown sugar
3/4 cup shortening
1 cup chopped walnuts
1 cup raisins

Sift the flour, cinnamon, baking soda and salt together and set aside. Beat the eggs, brown sugar and shortening in a mixer bowl. Add the flour mixture, walnuts and raisins and mix well. Drop by teaspoonfuls 3 inches apart onto a greased cookie sheet. Bake at 350 degrees for 10 minutes. Remove from the cookie sheet while still warm.

Yield: 5 dozen

Oatmeal Cookies

1 1/2 cups flour
1 teaspoon baking soda
1 teaspoon salt
1 cup butter, softened
1 cup sugar

1 cup packed brown sugar
2 eggs, beaten
3 cups quick-cooking oats
1/2 cup chopped pecans or walnuts
1 teaspoon vanilla extract

Mix the flour, baking soda and salt together and set aside. Cream the butter, sugar and brown sugar in a mixer bowl until light and fluffy. Beat in the eggs, then the oats. Add the flour mixture, pecans and vanilla and mix well. Chill slightly. Shape into 3 long narrow rolls on waxed paper. Freeze or chill for 1 hour or longer. Cut into slices and place on a cookie sheet. Bake at 375 degrees for 10 to 12 minutes or until lightly browned. Unbaked rolls may be frozen and sliced as needed.

Yield: 1 dozen

Orange Cookies

3¹/₂ cups flour
2 teaspoons baking powder
¹/₂ teaspoon salt
1 teaspoon baking soda
1 cup butter, softened

1¹/₂ cups packed brown sugar
2 eggs
Grated peel of 1 orange
1 cup buttermilk
Orange Frosting

Sift the flour, baking powder, salt and baking soda together and set aside. Beat the butter in a mixer bowl. Add the brown sugar gradually, beating constantly until light and fluffy. Add the eggs and orange peel and mix well. Add the flour mixture and buttermilk alternately, beating well after each addition. Drop by teaspoonfuls onto a greased cookie sheet. Bake at 375 degrees for 12 to 15 minutes. Spread Orange Frosting over the warm cookies.

Yield: 6 to 7 dozen

Orange Frosting

2 cups confectioners' sugar
¹/₄ cup orange juice

2 tablespoons butter, softened

Combine the confectioners' sugar, orange juice and butter in a mixer bowl and beat until of spreading consistency.

Sugar Cookies

2 cups sifted flour
1/2 teaspoon baking soda
1 teaspoon baking powder
1/2 cup shortening
1/2 teaspoon salt
1/2 teaspoon grated lemon peel

1/2 teaspoon nutmeg
1 cup sugar
2 eggs
2 tablespoons milk
Sugar to taste

Sift the flour, baking soda and baking powder together and set aside. Combine the shortening, salt, lemon peel, nutmeg, 1 cup sugar and eggs in a bowl and beat until smooth. Add the flour mixture and mix well. Stir in the milk. Drop by tablespoonfuls onto greased cookie sheets. Flatten with a 3-inch glass covered with a damp cloth. Sprinkle with additional sugar. Bake at 375 degrees for 8 to 10 minutes or until lightly browned.

Yield: 2 dozen

Martian Cookies

1 1/2 cups flour
1 teaspoon cinnamon
1/2 teaspoon baking soda
1/2 cup butter, softened
3/4 cup sugar
1 egg

1/2 teaspoon vanilla extract
1 cup quick-cooking oats
1 cup shredded unpeeled zucchini
1 cup chopped pecans or walnuts
1/2 cup chocolate chips
1/2 cup butterscotch chips

Beat the flour, cinnamon and baking soda at low speed in a medium mixer bowl until mixed. Beat the butter at medium speed in a large mixer bowl. Add the sugar gradually, beating constantly until light and fluffy. Beat in the egg and vanilla. Add the flour mixture gradually, beating well after each addition. Stir in the oats, zucchini, pecans, chocolate chips and butterscotch chips. Drop by rounded teaspoonfuls 2 inches apart onto nonstick cookie sheets. Bake at 350 degrees for 10 to 12 minutes or until golden brown. Cool on a wire rack.

Yield: 4 dozen

Grand Marnier Almond Brownies

1 cup butter
1 cup bittersweet chocolate
5 eggs
1¹/₂ cups sugar
2 teaspoons Grand Marnier

1 teaspoon grated orange peel
1 teaspoon vanilla extract
²/₃ cup toasted slivered almonds
²/₃ cup flour, sifted
¹/₂ cup raisins

Combine the butter and chocolate in a heavy medium saucepan. Cook over very low heat until melted, stirring constantly until smooth. Remove from the heat. Cool slightly.

Beat the eggs and sugar in a mixer bowl until blended and smooth. Stir in the Grand Marnier, orange peel and vanilla. Stir in the almonds, then the chocolate mixture. Fold in the flour. Fold in the raisins.

Spoon the batter into a lightly buttered and floured 9x13-inch baking pan. Bake at 350 degrees for 25 minutes or until the edges crack and a wooden pick inserted near the center comes out clean.

Cool in the pan on a wire rack for 30 minutes. Cut into squares. Remove the brownies to a wire rack to cool completely.

Yield: 16 servings

From the Heart...

"A volunteer is like a rare gem. When placed in the right setting and cared for, they will shine and give pleasure to all who see them."
—Unknown

...of Our House

Sinfully Rich Brownies

These are rich and fudgy brownies, but overbeating the batter will make them too cakelike.

5 ounces bittersweet chocolate
2/3 cup unsalted butter
4 small eggs
2 cups sugar
1½ cups flour
1 teaspoon baking powder

1 teaspoon salt
1 teaspoon almond extract
2 tablespoons vanilla extract
2 cups chocolate chips
1 (8-ounce) package coarsely
chopped walnuts

Combine the bittersweet chocolate and butter in a double boiler. Cook until melted, stirring constantly until blended and smooth. Remove from the heat. Cool slightly.

Combine the eggs and sugar in a bowl. Add the chocolate mixture and mix well. Blend in the flour, baking powder, salt, almond extract and vanilla extract; do not overbeat. Stir in the chocolate chips and walnuts.

Spread the batter in a buttered 8x8-inch baking pan. Bake at 350 degrees for 30 minutes or until the sides begin to pull away from the pan. Let cool before cutting into squares.

Yield: 8 to 12 servings

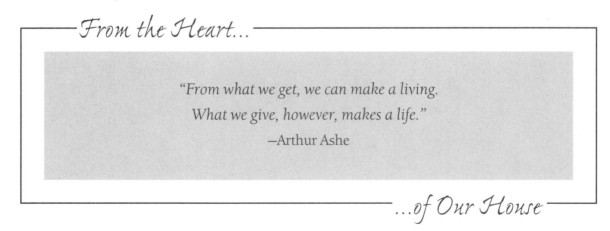

From the Heart...

"*From what we get, we can make a living.
What we give, however, makes a life.*"
—Arthur Ashe

...of Our House

Cherry Chewbilees

1¹/₄ cups flour
¹/₂ cup packed brown sugar
¹/₃ cup butter-flavor shortening
¹/₂ cup finely chopped walnuts
¹/₂ cup flaked coconut
16 ounces cream cheese, softened

²/₃ cup sugar
2 eggs
2 teaspoons vanilla extract
1 (21-ounce) can cherry pie filling
¹/₂ cup chopped walnuts

Grease a 9x13-inch baking pan with butter-flavor shortening. Combine the flour and brown sugar in a bowl and mix well. Cut in the shortening until crumbly. Stir in the walnuts and coconut. Remove and reserve ¹/₂ cup of the crumb mixture. Press the remaining crumb mixture over the bottom of the prepared baking pan. Bake at 350 degrees for 10 minutes or until lightly browned.

Beat the cream cheese, sugar, eggs and vanilla at medium speed in a small mixer bowl until blended and smooth. Spread over the hot crust. Bake for 15 minutes. Remove from the oven.

Spread the pie filling over the cream cheese layer. Mix the reserved crumb mixture and ¹/₂ cup walnuts in a bowl. Sprinkle over the pie filling. Bake for 15 minutes. Cool in the pan. Chill, covered, for several hours.

May instead be prepared in muffin cups. Decrease the last 2 baking times to 10 to 12 minutes each.

Yield: 36 servings

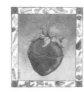

Apple Pie

1 (15-ounce) package all ready
pie pastries
³/₄ cup apple juice
³/₄ cup orange juice
³/₄ cup sugar
7 to 8 medium apples, peeled, cut into
¹/₂-inch wedges
¹/₄ cup apple juice
¹/₄ cup orange juice

¹/₄ cup cornstarch
1 tablespoon margarine or butter
¹/₈ teaspoon salt
¹/₄ teaspoon vanilla extract
¹/₂ cup whipping cream
2 tablespoons sugar
¹/₄ teaspoon vanilla extract
1 to 3 tablespoons chopped walnuts

Prepare the pie crust using the package directions for 1 unfilled pie crust in a 9-inch pie plate. Bake at 450 degrees for 9 to 11 minutes or until light golden brown. Cool completely.

Combine ³/₄ cup apple juice, ³/₄ cup orange juice and ³/₄ sugar in a large saucepan. Bring to a boil. Add the apple wedges. Cover and return to a boil; reduce the heat. Simmer, covered, for 3 to 5 minutes or just until the apples are tender-crisp. Remove the apples with a slotted spoon and set aside.

Blend ¹/₄ cup apple juice, ¹/₄ cup orange juice and cornstarch in a small bowl. Stir into the hot mixture in the saucepan. Cook over medium heat until the mixture thickens and boils, stirring constantly. Cook for 1 minute longer. Remove from the heat. Add the margarine, salt and ¹/₄ teaspoon vanilla and mix well. Remove from the heat. Cool for 10 minutes. Add the apples. Spoon the apple mixture into the baked crust. Chill for 3 hours or until set.

Beat the whipping cream in a mixer bowl until soft peaks form. Add 2 tablespoons sugar and ¹/₄ teaspoon vanilla gradually, beating constantly until stiff peaks form. Spread over the pie filling. Sprinkle with the walnuts.

Yield: 8 servings

French Silk Chocolate Pie

½ cup butter, softened
¾ cup sugar
1 ounce bittersweet chocolate, melted
1 teaspoon vanilla extract

2 eggs
1 baked (9-inch) pie shell
1 cup whipping cream, whipped
½ cup chopped walnuts (optional)

Cream the butter and sugar in a mixer bowl until light and fluffy. Blend in the chocolate and vanilla. Add the eggs 1 at a time, beating for 5 minutes after each addition. Spoon into the pie shell. Chill for 2 hours or longer. Top with the whipped cream. Sprinkle with the walnuts.

Yield: 8 servings

Lemonade Pie

1 (6-ounce) can frozen lemonade
concentrate, partially thawed
1 pint vanilla ice cream, softened

8 ounces whipped topping
1 graham cracker pie shell

Beat the lemonade concentrate at low speed in a mixer bowl for 30 seconds. Add the ice cream gradually, beating until blended. Fold in the whipped topping. Freeze until the mixture will mound. Spoon into the pie shell. Freeze for 4 hours to overnight. Let stand for 20 to 30 minutes before serving. Garnish with fresh strawberries.

Yield: 8 servings

Chocolate Linzer Tart

2 all ready pie pastries	1 egg
6 ounces semisweet chocolate	1 egg yolk
1/2 cup margarine or butter, softened	1 cup ground toasted almonds
1/2 cup sugar	1/2 cup seedless raspberry preserves

Fit 1 pastry into a 9-inch tart pan. Bake at 425 degrees for 5 to 8 minutes or until the crust begins to brown.

Combine the chocolate and 2 tablespoons of the margarine in a large microwave-safe bowl. Microwave on High for 2 minutes or until the margarine is melted. Stir until the chocolate is melted.

Cream the remaining 6 tablespoons margarine and sugar in a large mixer bowl until light and fluffy. Beat in 1 egg, 1 egg yolk and the almonds. Stir in the chocolate mixture. Spread evenly over the baked crust. Top with the preserves.

Cut the remaining pastry into 1/2-inch strips. Arrange lattice-fashion over the pie. Beat 1 egg white in a mixer bowl until foamy. Brush over the pastry strips.

Bake at 425 degrees for 10 minutes. Reduce the oven temperature to 350 degrees. Bake for 30 minutes or until the crust is golden brown. Cool on a wire rack.

Yield: 10 servings

White Chocolate Cheesecake with Cranberry Swirl

The recipe for this elegant dessert comes from a parish priest in Wisconsin who is justifiably famous for his cheesecakes.

1 (8-ounce) package
gingersnaps, ground
6 tablespoons melted butter
1½ teaspoons minced orange peel
1½ cups cranberries
¾ cup orange juice
¼ cup sugar
2 tablespoons cranberry or
orange liqueur

3 tablespoons dried currants
1 tablespoon grated orange peel
½ teaspoon ground cinnamon
6 ounces white chocolate,
finely chopped
24 ounces cream cheese, softened
¾ cup sugar
4 large eggs
White chocolate curls or shavings

Mix the ground gingersnaps, butter and minced orange peel in a medium bowl. Press the crumb mixture over the bottom and 2 inches up the side of a springform pan. Combine the cranberries, orange juice, ¼ cup sugar, liqueur, currants, grated orange peel and cinnamon in a small heavy saucepan. Simmer over medium heat for 8 minutes or until the cranberries lose their shape and the mixture is slightly thickened, stirring occasionally. Remove to a food processor container. Process until smooth. Strain the mixture and let cool. Chill, covered, until needed. Heat the white chocolate in a double boiler over simmering water until melted, stirring until smooth. Cool slightly.

For the filling, beat the cream cheese in a large mixer bowl until smooth. Stir in ¾ cup sugar. Add the eggs 1 at a time, beating well after each addition. Add the white chocolate gradually, mixing well after each addition. Spoon half the filling into the springform pan. Drop half the cranberry mixture 2 tablespoonfuls at a time over the filling, spacing evenly. Swirl the cranberry mixture through the filling with a small sharp knife. Repeat with the remaining filling and cranberry mixture. Bake at 350 degrees for 40 minutes or until the edge of the cheesecake is puffed and golden brown; the center will not be set. Cool on a wire rack. Chill overnight. Loosen the edge of the cheesecake from the pan with a small sharp knife. Remove the side of the pan. Press white chocolate curls around the edge of the cheesecake.

Yield: 10 servings

Apple and Oat Pudding

$^{1}/_{2}$ cup quick-cooking rolled oats
$^{1}/_{2}$ cup flour
$^{1}/_{4}$ cup melted butter or margarine
2$^{1}/_{2}$ cups sliced peeled apples

$^{1}/_{2}$ teaspoon cinnamon
$^{1}/_{2}$ cup maple syrup
Whipped cream or whipped topping

Mix the oats, flour and butter in a bowl until crumbly. Arrange the apples in a greased 8x8-inch baking dish. Sprinkle with the cinnamon. Spoon the syrup over the top. Sprinkle with the crumb mixture. Bake, covered with foil, at 375 degrees for 35 minutes. Bake, uncovered, for 10 minutes or until browned. Spoon into 4 dessert dishes. Serve hot with whipped cream. May instead be covered with plastic wrap and microwaved for 16 minutes, turning once. Recipe may be doubled or tripled.

Yield: 4 servings

Old-Fashioned Baked Custard

6 eggs
$^{1}/_{2}$ teaspoon salt
$^{2}/_{3}$ cup sugar

3 cups scalded milk
1 teaspoon vanilla extract
Nutmeg to taste

Beat the eggs, salt and sugar lightly in a mixer bowl. Beat in the milk gradually, stirring until the sugar is dissolved. Add the vanilla. Spoon into a buttered baking dish or individual custard cups. Sprinkle with nutmeg. Set the baking dish in a larger pan. Add enough water to the pan to come halfway up the sides of the baking dish. Bake at 300 to 325 degrees for 1 hour or until a knife inserted near the center comes out clean.

Yield: 8 servings

Tiramisù

1 pint whipping cream
¼ cup confectioners' sugar
17 ounces mascarpone
cheese, softened
2½ cups brewed espresso
1 tablespoon sugar

2 tablespoons brandy
1½ teaspoons brandy extract
2 (7-ounce) packages
Italian ladyfingers
Sugar-free cocoa mix

Beat the whipping cream in a mixer bowl until soft peaks form. Beat in the confectioners' sugar and mascarpone cheese. Set aside.

Pour the espresso into a shallow bowl or pie plate. Add the sugar, brandy and brandy extract. Dip one side of each ladyfinger quickly into the espresso mixture, preparing enough to line the bottom of an 8x11-inch glass baking dish. Arrange the ladyfingers dry side down in the baking dish. Cover with ⅓ of the cream mixture. Dip both sides of enough ladyfingers for 1 layer in the espresso mixture. Place in the baking dish and top with ⅓ of the cream mixture. Repeat with another layer of ladyfingers and the remaining cream mixture. Sprinkle with the cocoa mix. Chill, covered with plastic wrap, for 8 hours or longer.

Yield: 12 to 15 servings

From the Heart...

"I feel the greatest award for doing is the opportunity to do more."
–Jonas Salk, M.D.

...of Our House

$\mathcal{B}$lueberry Crisp

3 cups blueberries
2 tablespoons lemon juice
2/3 cup packed brown sugar
1/2 cup flour

1/2 cup quick-cooking oats
1/3 cup butter, softened
3/4 teaspoon cinnamon
1/4 teaspoon salt

Arrange the blueberries in an 8x8-inch baking dish. Sprinkle with the lemon juice. Mix the brown sugar, flour, oats, butter, cinnamon and salt in a bowl. Sprinkle over the blueberries. Bake at 375 degrees for 30 minutes or until the topping is browned and the dessert is heated through. May instead be microwaved for 12 to 14 minutes.

Yield: 6 servings

$\mathcal{S}$trawberries Nirope

2 pints large strawberries
1 (4-ounce) package vanilla instant
pudding mix

1 cup milk
2 teaspoons almond extract
1 cup whipping cream, whipped

Wash the strawberries and cut off the stem ends so that the strawberries can stand. Make an X-shaped cut in the top of each strawberry, cutting to but not through the bottom. Push open gently; set aside. Beat the pudding mix and milk in a mixer bowl. Add the almond extract. Fold in the whipped cream. Spoon into a decorator tube or bag fitted with a star tip. Pipe the whipped cream mixture into the centers of the strawberries. Chill until serving time.

Yield: 8 servings

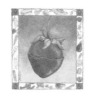

*B*aklava

3 cups sugar
2 cups water
1 cinnamon stick
Juice of ¹/₂ lemon
1 pound walnuts, finely chopped
¹/₃ cup sugar

¹/₂ teaspoon cinnamon
¹/₄ teaspoon ground cloves
¹/₄ teaspoon nutmeg
1 (16-ounce) package phyllo
1 pound unsalted butter, melted

Combine 3 cups sugar, water, cinnamon stick and lemon juice in a saucepan. Boil gently for 20 minutes or to 230 degrees on a candy thermometer. Set aside to cool. Remove and discard the cinnamon stick.

Combine the walnuts, ¹/₃ cup sugar, ¹/₂ teaspoon cinnamon, cloves and nutmeg in a bowl and mix well; set aside. Butter a 9x13-inch baking pan. Trim the phyllo to fit the pan.

Place 6 sheets of the phyllo in the pan, brushing each sheet generously with butter. Sprinkle evenly with a thin layer of the walnut mixture. Cover with 4 buttered phyllo sheets. Sprinkle with a thin layer of the walnut mixture. Repeat this process until all the phyllo sheets and walnut mixture are used, using 8 sheets of phyllo for the top layer. Cut into diamond shapes.

Bake at 325 degrees for 30 minutes. Reduce the oven temperature to 300 degrees. Bake for 30 minutes or until golden brown. Pour the cooled syrup over the hot baklava. Let stand overnight before serving.

Editor's Note: Because phyllo dries out quickly, do not open the package until the other ingredients are at hand. Keep the unused sheets covered with waxed paper topped with a damp towel until needed. It will not matter if each layer does not fit perfectly into the pan.

Yield: 24 servings

Index

Accompaniments
Mango Chutney, 131
Pear Chutney, 112

Appetizers
Apple Pizza, 19
Asparagus Treats, 19
Baked Brie and Brandied
    Mushrooms, 18
Chile Pepper Pie, 21
Clams Casino, 20
Lemon Chicken, 23
Mushroom Palmiers, 24
Pepperoni and Cheese Puffs, 20
Southwest Appetizer Cheesecake, 22
Vegetable Squares, 21

Apples
Apple and Oat Pudding, 168
Apple Pie, 164
Apple Pizza, 19
Pork Cutlets with Apples, Parsnips and
    Cabbage, 115
Purée of Butternut Squash and Apple
    Soup, 52
Scalloped Sweet Potatoes and
    Apples, 145

Artichokes
Cream of Artichoke Soup, 49
Hot Artichoke Dip, 13

Asparagus
Asparagus Bundles with Prosciutto, 135
Asparagus Soup, 50
Asparagus Treats, 19
Asparagus with Lemon Vinaigrette, 136

Beans
Bristol's Best Baked Beans, 137
Orecchiette with Cauliflower, Potatoes
    and Kidney Beans, 70

Beef
Beef Bourguignon, 103

Beef Fillets with Mozzarella Cheese, 104
Mushroom and Spinach-Stuffed Beef
    Tenderloin, 101
Roast Beef Salad with Pesto Vinaigrette, 61
Sliced Steak with Mustard Sauce, 102
Texas Chili, 56

Beverages
Hot Buttered Sherry, 27
Mint Cooler, 25
Old New England Hot Mulled
    Punch, 27
Raspberry Slush, 25
Sophisticated Strawberry Shakes, 26
Strawberry Smoothie, 26

Blueberries
Blueberry Crisp, 170
Blueberry Tea Cake, 31

Breads
Banana Buttermilk Buckwheat
    Pancakes, 37
Biscotti, 39
Blueberry Tea Cake, 31
Bran Muffins, 36
Crepes Stuffed with Ricotta Cheese and
    Prosciutto, 38
Garlic Bread, 32
Johnnycakes, 43
Lemon Bread, 33
New England Brown Bread, 32
Nirope Nut Bread, 34
Strawberry Brunch Loaf, 35

Brownies
Grand Marnier Almond Brownies, 161
Sinfully Rich Brownies, 162

Cabbage
Pork Cutlets with Apples, Parsnips and
    Cabbage, 115
Spinach and Cabbage Salad with
    Pecans, 59
Summertime Coleslaw, 57

Cakes
Carrot Cake with Cream Cheese
    Frosting, 153
Chocolate Fudge Cake with Fudge
    Frosting, 154
Hummingbird Cake, 156
Pumpkin Chocolate Chip Cake, 156
White Chocolate Cake, 155

Carrots
Carrot Cake with Cream Cheese
    Frosting, 153
Carrot Casserole, 139
Carrot Raisin Salad, 58
Copper Carrots, 138

Chicken
Almond Chicken, 128
Baked Chicken Breasts with Gruyère
    Cheese and Mushrooms, 122
Bleu Cheese-Stuffed Chicken, 124
Chicken Cordon Bleu, 126
Chicken Dijon, 121
Chicken Marsala, 123
Chicken Mexicana, 119
Chicken with Penne, 79
Company Chicken, 120
Lemon Chicken, 23
Roasted Chicken with Peppers and
    Potatoes, 118
South County Chicken Pie, 127
Stir-Fry Chicken, 125
White Chili, 55

Clams
Cardi's Clams and Spaghetti, 81
Clams Casino, 20
Linguini in White Clam Sauce, 67

Cookies
Apricot Slices, 157
Cherry Chewbilees, 163
Hermits, 158
Martian Cookies, 160
Oatmeal Cookies, 158

Orange Cookies, 159
Sugar Cookies, 160

Crab Meat
Crab Dip, 14
Sherried Crab Quiche, 42

Desserts
Apple and Oat Pudding, 168
Baklava, 171
Blueberry Crisp, 170
Old-Fashioned Baked Custard, 168
Strawberries Nirope, 170
Tiramisù, 169
White Chocolate Cheesecake with
    Cranberry Swirl, 167

Dips
Crab Dip, 14
Hot Artichoke Dip, 13
Hot Fresh Salsa, 16
Hummus-Style Dip, 15
Mustard Dill Dip, 13

Egg Dishes
Company Eggs, 40
Eggs Rustica, 40
Spinach Frittata, 41

Eggplant
Baked Eggplant and
    Feta Cheese, 140
Eggplant Turkey Casserole, 129

Fish
Cajun Cod, 85
Scrod Imperial, 86
Tangy Seafood Kabobs, 94

Frostings/Glazes
Cream Cheese Frosting, 153
Fudge Frosting, 154
Lemon Glaze, 33
Orange Frosting, 159
White Chocolate Frosting, 155

Ground Beef
French Meat Pie, 105
Kids' Kasserole, 106
Nirope Vegetable Soup, 54

Ham
Asparagus Bundles with Prosciutto, 135
Crepes Stuffed with Ricotta Cheese and
    Prosciutto, 38
Due Fettuccini with Prosciutto, 76
Grilled Shrimp with Prosciutto and
    Basil, 93

Lamb
Lamb with Garlic and Rosemary, 109
Mediterranean Lamb Chops, 110

Lobster
Creamed Lobster and Johnnycakes, 43
Easy Lobster Newburg, 87
Venus de Milo Lobster Casserole, 88

Marinades
Garlic Basil Marinade, 83
Teriyaki Marinade, 83

Mushrooms
Baked Brie and Brandied
    Mushrooms, 18
Baked Chicken Breasts with Gruyère
    Cheese and Mushrooms, 122
Corn and Mushroom Bake, 139
Mushroom and Spinach-Stuffed Beef
    Tenderloin, 101
Mushroom Palmiers, 24
Sausage and Mushrooms with Creamy
    Polenta, 117
Sautéed Spinach with Shiitake
    Mushrooms, 142
Seared Scallops with Wild
    Mushrooms, 89
Veal Scaloppine with Mushrooms, 108

Pasta
Baked Ditali with Sweet and Hot Italian
    Sausages, 77
Baked Ziti with Spinach and
    Tomatoes, 78
Cardi's Clams and Spaghetti, 81
Chicken with Penne, 79
Creamy Spinach and Tortellini, 73
Due Fettuccini with Prosciutto, 76
Linguini à la Nirope, 68
Linguini in White Clam Sauce, 67
Macaroni and Cheese for Grownups, 69

Orecchiette with Cauliflower, Potatoes
    and Kidney Beans, 70
Pasta Carbonara, 75
Pasta Providence, 72
Pasta Salad with Red Wine
    Vinaigrette, 60
Penne, Pepper and Salmon in Garlic
    Sauce, 80
Perciatelli with Greens and Seasoned
    Bread Crumbs, 71
Scampi Fettuccini with Garlic and
    Olive Oil, 82
Vermicelli with Lemony Green
    Vegetables, 74

Pies
Apple Pie, 164
Chocolate Linzer Tart, 166
French Silk Chocolate Pie, 165
Lemonade Pie, 165

Pork
Cajun-Style Pork Chops, 114
Crown Roast of Pork with Apricot
    Bread Stuffing, 111
French Meat Pie, 105
Marinated Pork Tenderloins with
    Sour Cream Mustard Sauce, 113
Pasta Carbonara, 75
Pork Cutlets with Apples, Parsnips and
    Cabbage, 115
Pork with Pear Chutney, 112
Raspberry Pork Chops, 116

Potatoes
Dijonnaise Potatoes, 141
Grilled New Potatoes, 141
Orecchiette with Cauliflower, Potatoes
    and Kidney Beans, 70
Roasted Chicken with Peppers and
    Potatoes, 118

Quiches
Sherried Crab Quiche, 42
Tomato Mozzarella Tart, 45

Raspberries
Raspberry Pork Chops, 116
Raspberry Slush, 25
Raspberry Vinaigrette, 63

Rice
Buttered Baked Rice, 148
Italian Rice and Spinach, 148
Risotto with Smoked Mozzarella and
  Escarole, 149
Shrimp and Rice Salad, 62

Salad Dressings
Herbal Vinaigrette, 62
Italian Salad Dressing, 63
Lemon Dressing, 23
Lemon Vinaigrette, 136
Pesto Vinaigrette, 61
Raspberry Vinaigrette, 63
Red Wine Vinaigrette, 60

Salads
Carrot Raisin Salad, 58
Lentil Salad, 58
Pasta Salad with Red Wine Vinaigrette, 60
Roast Beef Salad with Pesto
  Vinaigrette, 61
Shrimp and Rice Salad, 62
Spinach and Cabbage Salad with
  Pecans, 59
Summertime Coleslaw, 57

Salmon
Grilled Salmon, 83
Penne, Pepper and Salmon in Garlic
  Sauce, 80
Salmon with Dijon Sauce, 84

Sauces
Creamy Basil Sauce, 96
Creamy Dill Sauce, 44
Dijon Sauce, 84
Garlic Sauce, 80
Lemon Pepper Sauce, 120
Mayor Vincent A. Cianci, Jr.'s Marinara
  Sauce, 97
Mustard Sauce, 102
Pesto, 96
Sour Cream Mustard Sauce, 113
Sun-Dried Tomato Sauce, 97
Szechuan Peanut Sauce, 131
Tomato Sauce, 107

Sausage
Baked Ditali with Sweet and Hot Italian
  Sausages, 77

Pepperoni and Cheese Puffs, 20
Sausage and Mushrooms with Creamy
  Polenta, 117

Scallops
Scallops Nantucket, 90
Seared Scallops with Wild
  Mushrooms, 89
Tangy Seafood Kabobs, 94

Shrimp
Grilled Shrimp with Prosciutto and
  Basil, 93
Linguini à la Nirope, 68
Scampi Fettuccini with Garlic and
  Olive Oil, 82
Shrimp and Rice Salad, 62
Shrimp with Creamy Dill Sauce, 44
Shrimp with Feta Cheese, 95
Stir-Fried Shrimp with Ginger and
  Garlic, 92
Tangy Seafood Kabobs, 94
Teriyaki Shrimp, 91

Soups/Stews
Asparagus Soup, 50
Basic Vegetable Stock, 146
Cream of Artichoke Soup, 49
Farmer's Fresh Tomato Soup, 53
New England Cheddar
  Cheese Soup, 51
Nirope Vegetable Soup, 54
Purée of Butternut Squash and Apple
  Soup, 52
Texas Chili, 56
White Chili, 55

Spinach
Baked Ziti with Spinach and
  Tomatoes, 78
Creamy Spinach and Tortellini, 73
Italian Rice and Spinach, 148
Mushroom and Spinach-Stuffed Beef
  Tenderloin, 101
Quick-and-Easy Sicilian
  Spinach, 143
Sautéed Spinach with Shiitake
  Mushrooms, 142
Spinach and Cabbage Salad with
  Pecans, 59
Spinach Frittata, 41

Spreads
Herbed Cream Cheese, 16
Olive Nut Spread, 17
Swiss Cheese Spread, 17

Squash
Purée of Butternut Squash and Apple
  Soup, 52
Squash Soufflé, 143

Strawberries
Sophisticated Strawberry Shakes, 26
Strawberries Nirope, 170
Strawberry Brunch Loaf, 35
Strawberry Smoothie, 26

Sweet Potatoes
Scalloped Sweet Potatoes and
  Apples, 145
Sweet Potato Streusel Casserole, 144

Tomatoes
Baked Ziti with Spinach and
  Tomatoes, 78
Farmer's Fresh Tomato Soup, 53
Mayor Vincent A. Cianci, Jr.'s Marinara
  Sauce, 97
Sun-Dried Tomato Sauce, 97
Tomato Mozzarella Tart, 45
Tomato Sauce, 107

Turkey
Barley and Turkey Stuffed Peppers, 130
Eggplant Turkey Casserole, 129

Veal
Veal Parmigiana, 107
Veal Scaloppine with Mushrooms, 108

Vegetables
Beets with Orange Sauce, 138
Cold Weather Roasted Vegetables, 147
Julienned Vegetables, 146
Lemon Vegetables, 145
Lentil Salad, 58
Nirope Vegetable Soup, 54
Orecchiette with Cauliflower, Potatoes
  and Kidney Beans, 70
Vegetable Squares, 21
Vermicelli with Lemony Green
  Vegetables, 74

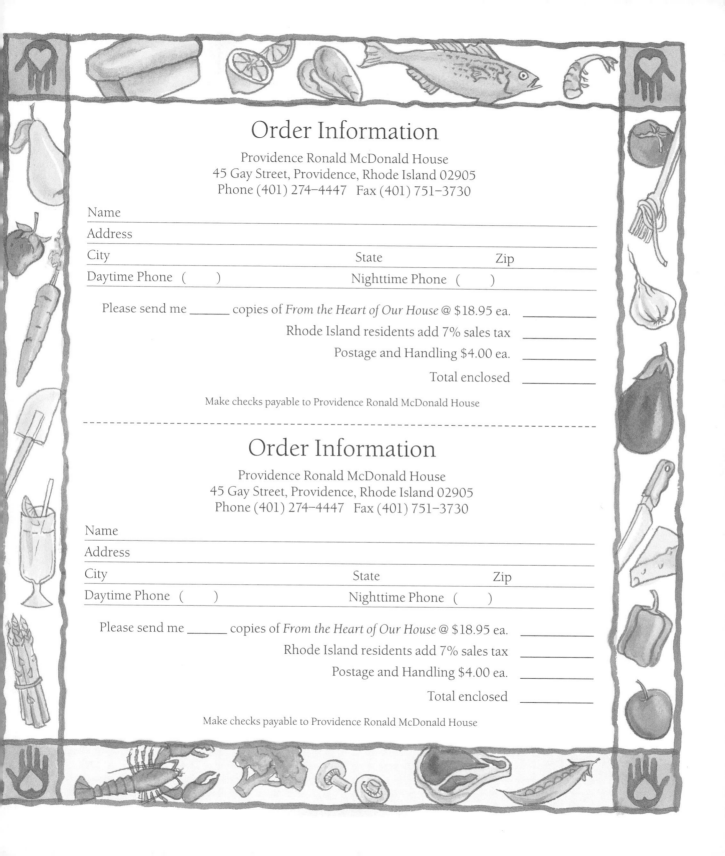

Order Information

Providence Ronald McDonald House
45 Gay Street, Providence, Rhode Island 02905
Phone (401) 274–4447 Fax (401) 751–3730

Name

Address

City   State   Zip

Daytime Phone (   )   Nighttime Phone (   )

Please send me _____ copies of *From the Heart of Our House* @ $18.95 ea. _____

Rhode Island residents add 7% sales tax _____

Postage and Handling $4.00 ea. _____

Total enclosed _____

Make checks payable to Providence Ronald McDonald House

Order Information

Providence Ronald McDonald House
45 Gay Street, Providence, Rhode Island 02905
Phone (401) 274–4447 Fax (401) 751–3730

Name

Address

City   State   Zip

Daytime Phone (   )   Nighttime Phone (   )

Please send me _____ copies of *From the Heart of Our House* @ $18.95 ea. _____

Rhode Island residents add 7% sales tax _____

Postage and Handling $4.00 ea. _____

Total enclosed _____

Make checks payable to Providence Ronald McDonald House